KEY TO CHART USE

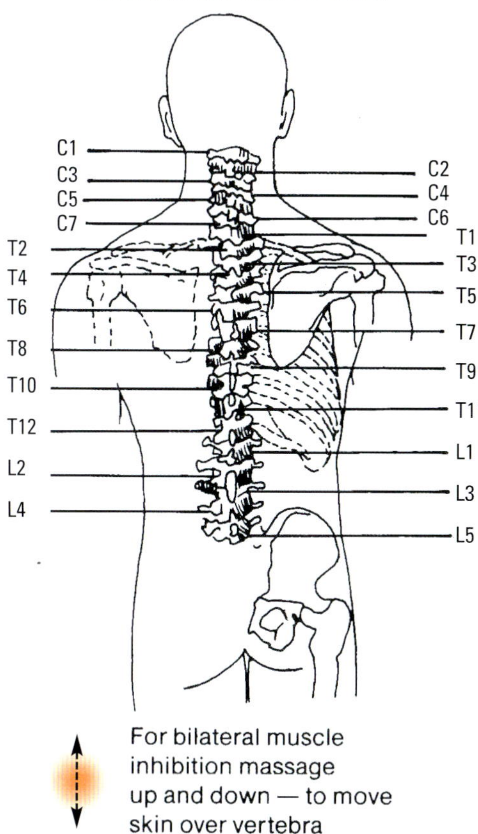

For bilateral muscle inhibition massage up and down — to move skin over vertebra

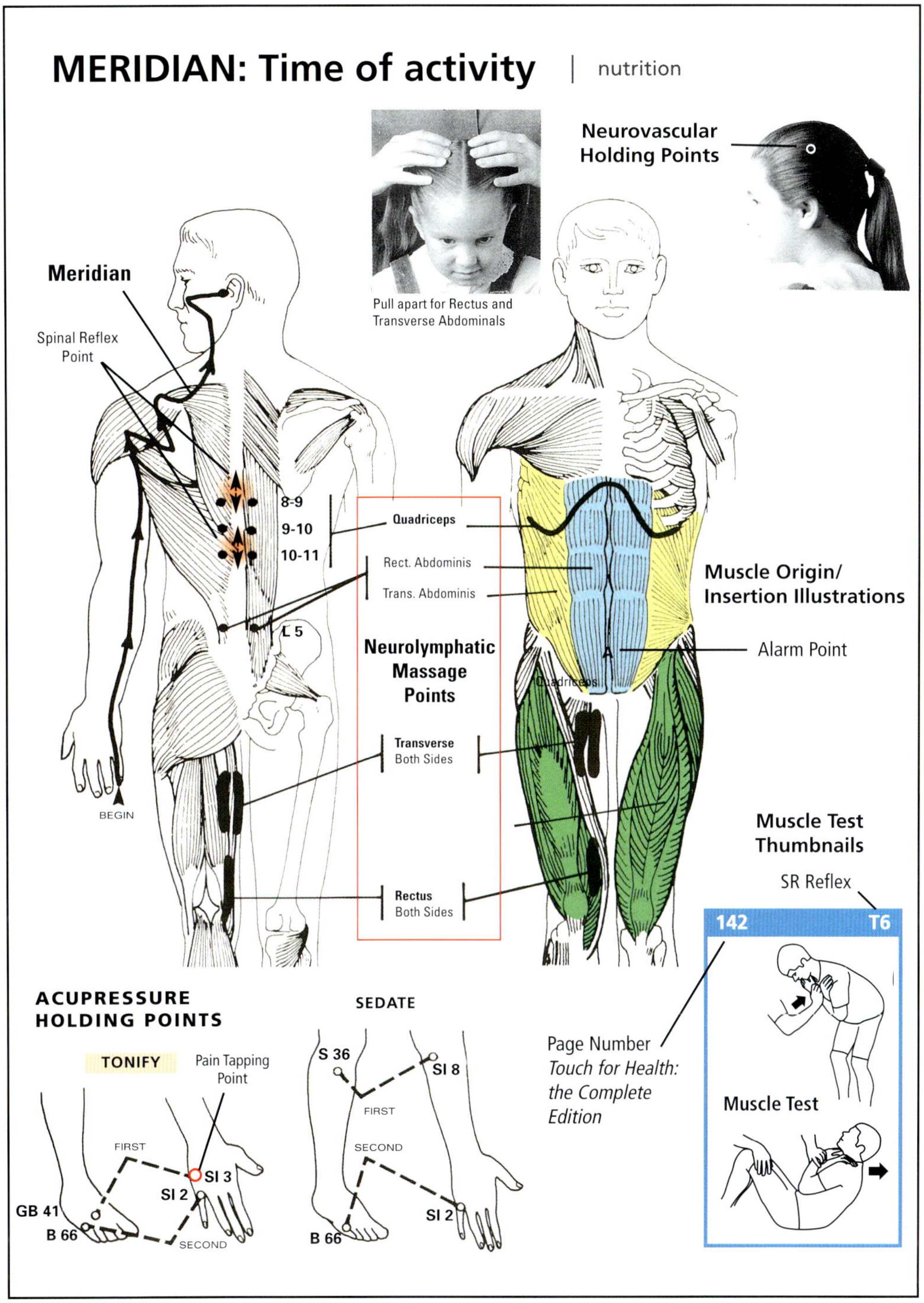

MERIDIAN: Time of activity | nutrition

Neurovascular Holding Points

Pull apart for Rectus and Transverse Abdominals

Meridian

Spinal Reflex Point

BEGIN

8-9

9-10

10-11

L 5

Neurolymphatic Massage Points

Quadriceps

Rect. Abdominis

Trans. Abdominis

Transverse Both Sides

Rectus Both Sides

Muscle Origin/ Insertion Illustrations

Alarm Point

Quadriceps

Muscle Test Thumbnails

SR Reflex

142 T6

Muscle Test

Page Number *Touch for Health: the Complete Edition*

ACUPRESSURE HOLDING POINTS

TONIFY

Pain Tapping Point

FIRST

SECOND

GB 41

B 66

SI 2

SI 3

SEDATE

S 36

SI 8

FIRST

SECOND

B 66

SI 2

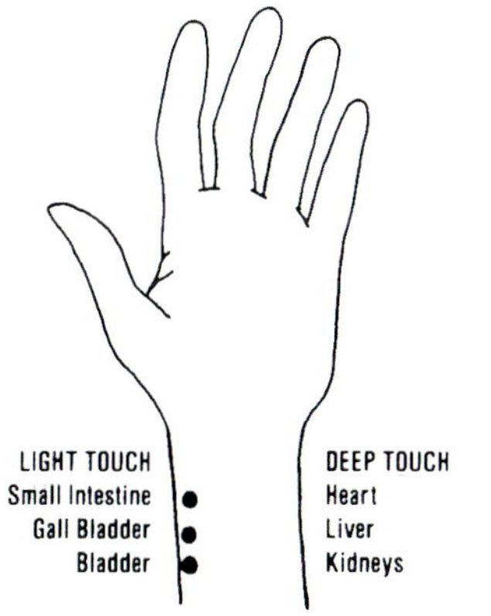

Light holding at Neurovascular/ AHP Points

Firm massage at Neurolymphatic points

Trace meridian beginning to end

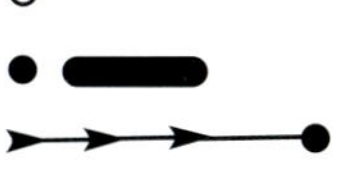

Pulse Points: CL for Over-Energy

RIGHT HAND

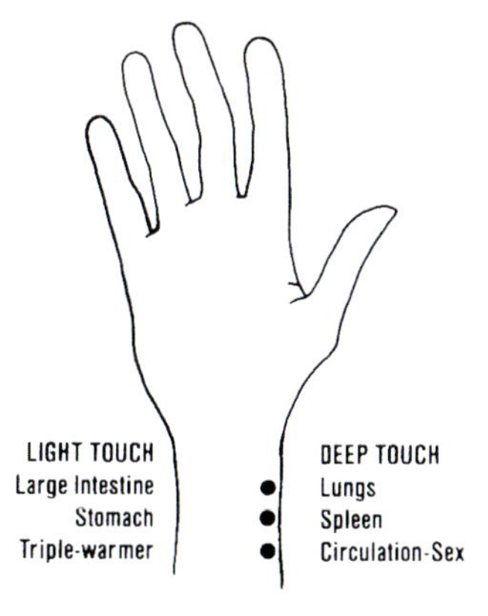

LEFT HAND

LIGHT TOUCH
Small Intestine
Gall Bladder
Bladder

DEEP TOUCH
Heart
Liver
Kidneys

For more information, see "Touch for Health: Complete Edition" by Dr. John & Matthew Thie and "eTouch", the electronic companion to Touch for Health, with over 101 animations.

OPTIONS FOR USING TOUCH FOR HEALTH

Goal Setting/ Goal Balancing

The TFH balance is more than just a structural balancing of the muscles. The muscles also give us an indication of balance and flow in the meridian energy system and the overall functioning of the person in their current life context. For each goal, there is a different pattern of energy blocks/ imbalance as indicated by the muscle tests. When we balance for a particular goal, the subsequent shifts in posture, attitude and energy can be profound and dramatic. Your goal can be as simple as improving your energy balance and enhancing your sense of Wellness, or it can be related to pain, symptoms, etc. It is MOST powerful if it is framed in terms of a positive outcome that you whole-heartedly want: improved range of motion, physical performance, personal best in an exam, a job interview, etc.

- Do any pre-checks you normally do.
- Frame your goal as a positive statement in present time.
- Measure your subjective feeling about the goal, and any pain/symptoms on an analog scale 0-10 (0 being NO pain, or no confidence in your goal, 10 being maximum pain, or optimum performance).
- Find the Five Element emotion related to the goal using the IM (Indicator Muscle): (Wood:Anger/Resentment, Fire: Joy, Earth: Sympathy/Empathy, Metal: Grief/Regret, Water: Fear/Anxiety).
- State your goal and simultaneously test the IM. The unlocking IM indicates stress related to the goal. If the IM does not unlock, make sure you are "present". You may need to rephrase your goal or think of a particular aspect to find an indicator muscle change. Now all of the subsequent muscle testing and balancing relates to the stated goal in mind.
- After balancing all of the muscles/meridians the IM should now lock. If there is still stress on the goal use Emotional Stress Release (ESR: light holding on the forehead)

OPTIONS FOR BALANCING: Cross-Referenced, TFH Complete Edition

See also DATABASE on page 36.

TFH Topic/Technique	TFH: Complete
TFH LEVEL I: Balancing-as-you-go	
Permission/Education	19-20; 22; 68
Posture Awareness	26-29
Zip Up, Switch On & Tune In	36-39
Muscle Testing, Accurate Indicator Muscle (AIM)	16-24, 41-47
*Unexpected Muscle Response	43
Pretests: (AIM, Water, Central Meridian, Switching) Physical, Emotional, and Energetic Challenges	41-47
Emotional Stress Release for Present Distress, Physical (or Emotional) Pain	38-40
Basic Goal-Setting/Balancing	72-73; 87-89
14-Muscle Balancing-as-you-go	68-78
MUSCLE/ENERGY BALANCING REFLEXES	
Spinal Reflex-SR (skin stretch), Neurolymphatic Massage Points (Firm Pressure), Neurovascular Holding Points (LIGHT holding), Meridian Tracing (trace within 3 "), Origin and Insertion Technique (Jiggling)/ Heavy Pressure	47-57,86,276
Challenging: (CL to Challenge a reflex)	59-62
Strengthening with Food; Balancing for Digestion	64, 299; 273
Walking, Cross Crawl	264-265
Auricular Energy, Visual Inhibition	251-252
*Opposing Muscle Strengthening; "Test Also" Muscles**	5, 277; 65
Surrogate Testing	256
Simple Pain Control: Feathering, Spindling: Flushing/Running Meridians	272-275
TFH LEVEL II: Assessment/1-Point Balancing	
28/14+ Muscle Balancing	69-78
MORE MUSCLE/ENERGY BALANCING REFLEXES	
Origin/Insertion (O/I): Spindle Cell, Golgi Tendon, Acupressure Holding Pts (AHP); Cerebro-Spinal Reflex	57-58, 84; 65
Circuit Locating (CL): switching, Reflex points	63, 233-235

TFH Topic/Technique (Level II continued)	TFH: Complete
Yin/Yang Concept	30
Assessment Balancing/1-Point Balancing	232-244
Alarm Points for Over-energy	58
24 Hour Wheel; 5 Elements	236-238; 240-244
ESR for Future Performance	258-259
Meridian Massage/Meridian Dance	34-35; 273&275
Meridian Walking	280
Basic Food Testing; Food Testing with C1 (Sensivity Mode)	301-302
More Simple Pain Control	272-275
*Sedating/ Re-strengthening a Muscle**	278
Cross Crawl Integration	266-267
Time of Day Balance	274-275

TOUCH FOR HEALTH METAPHORS WORKSHOP

Metaphor Balancing: Muscles, Meridians, 5-Elements, Food	66,67; 215-223
Fishing for Issues	308
Attractor Value	312

SEE ALSO: TFH Pocketbook, with Chinese Five Element Metaphors.

TFH Level III Reactive Muscles/Assessment Balancing Review

14/28/42 or 14+ muscle balancing	69, 77, 90-93
Color Balance	75, 262
Goal w/ 5 Element Emotions	74
Reactive Pattern Shortcut	293
Reactivity, Circuit Retaining Mode	290-298
Gait Testing and Balancing	268-271
ESR for Past Trauma; Past Balancing	259; 260
Sedation Techniques; Pain Tapping; Pulse Points	278-279; 280-281; 70
5-Element Balancing with Food; Foods for Balancing	302 ; 64
*Metaphorical/Symbolic Value of Food**	323

TFH Level IV : Postural Analysis; 42 muscles lying or standing; Review

42/ 14+ Muscle Balancing; Anatomical balancing	69-78; 283-284,286, 288-289/344
ESR with 5 Element Emotion	261
Sound Balance	75, 263
Luo Points	248-249
Figure Eight Energy	254-255
NL- Release	52
Postural Stress Relief	260-261
Posture Analysis	283-291
*Repeated Testing & Restrengthening with SR and NL**	276
*In-Depth Interview for Pain Control; In-Depth Interview for Remembering Wellness with Goal-Setting**	324-329;

* **Extra techniques in Complete Edition *not in regular IKC Syllabus***
See also DATABASE at end of book on page 36.

OPTIONS

MUSCLE REFERENCE BY MUSCLE

Muscle	Page*	Folio Page	Spinal Reflex Pt	Meridian Pain Tap	Meridian/Related Organ	Element	Peak Time
Abdominals: Rectus Abdominis	142	19	T6	SI3	SI/Small Intestine	FIRE	2:00 PM
Abdominals: Transverse/Oblique	143	19	T6	SI3	SI/Small Intestine	FIRE	2:00 PM
Adductors	172	25	L1	CX9	CX/Sex, Pericardium	FIRE	8:00 PM
Anterior Deltoid	196	29	T4	GB43	GB/Gallbladder	WOOD	12:00 mid
Anterior Serratus	212	33	T3 T4	LU10	LU/Lungs	METAL	4:00 AM
Brachioradialis	116	13	T12	S41	ST/Stomach	EARTH	8:00 AM
Coracobrachialis	214	33	T3 T4	LU10	LU/Lungs	METAL	4:00 AM
Deltoids	216	33	T2 T3	LU10	LU/Lungs	METAL	4:00 AM
Diaphragm	218	33	T12	LU10	LU/Lungs	METAL	4:00 AM
Fascia Lata	224	35	L2	LI11	LI/Large Intestine	METAL	6:00 AM
Gastrocnemius	190	27	T11 T12	TW3	TW/Adrenals	FIRE	10:00 PM
Gluteus Maximus	176	25	C2	CX9	CX/Sex, Pericardium	FIRE	8:00 PM
Gluteus Medius	170	25	L5	CX9	CX/Sex, Pericardium	FIRE	8:00 PM
Gracilis	186	27	T12	TW3	TW/Adrenals	FIRE	10:00 PM
Hamstrings	226	35	L4 L5	LI11	LI/Large Intestine	METAL	6:00 AM
Iliacus	164	23	T11	K7	K/Ileo-Cecal Valve	WATER	6:00 PM
Latissimus Dorsi	122	15	T7	SP2	SP/Pancreas	EARTH	10:00 AM
Levator Scapulae	112	13	C5 T8	S41	ST/Stomach	EARTH	8:00 AM
Lower Trapezius	124	15	T6	SP2	SP/Spleen	EARTH	10:00 AM
Middle Trapezius	124	15	T5 T6	SP2	SP/Spleen	EARTH	10:00 AM
Neck: Anterior Flexors	114	13	C2	S41	ST/Sinuses	EARTH	8:00 AM
Neck: Posterior Extensors	114	13	C2	S41	ST/Sinuses	EARTH	8:00 AM
Opponens Pollicis Longus	126	15	C4	SP2	SP/Spleen	EARTH	10:00 AM
Pectoralis Major Clavicular	110	13	T5	S41	ST/Stomach	EARTH	8:00 AM
Pectoralis Major Sternal	204	31	T5	LV8	LV/Liver	WOOD	2:00 AM
Peroneus	150	21	T12	BL67	BL/Bladder	WATER	4:00 PM
Piriformis	174	25	S1	CX9	CX/Sex, Pericardium	FIRE	8:00 PM
Popliteus	198	29	T12	GB43	GB/Gallbladder	WOOD	12:00 mid
Psoas	160	23	T12	K7	K/Kidneys	WATER	6:00 PM
Quadratus Lumborum	228	35	L4 L5	LI11	LI/Spine	METAL	6:00 AM
Quadriceps	140	19	T10	SI3	SI/Small Intestine	FIRE	2:00 PM
Rhomboids	206	31	T5	LV8	LV/Liver	WOOD	2:00 AM
Sacrospinalis	152	21	T12	BL67	BL/Bladder	WATER	4:00 PM
Sartorius	184	27	T11	TW3	TW/Adrenals	FIRE	10:00 PM
Soleus	188	27	T11 T12	TW3	TW/Adrenals	FIRE	10:00 PM
Subscapularis	134	17	T2	H9	H/Heart	FIRE	12:00 noon
Supraspinatus	98	11	C1 C2	NONE	C/Brain	GLOBAL	Night
Teres Major	104	11	T2	NONE	G/Spine	GLOBAL	Day
Teres Minor	182	27	T2	TW3	TW/Thyroid	FIRE	10:00 PM
Tibials: Anterior/Posterior	154	21	L5	BL67	BL/Bladder	WATER	4:00 PM
Triceps	128	15	T1	SP2	SP/Pancreas	EARTH	10:00 AM
Upper Trapezius	162	23	C7	K7	K/Eyes & Ears	WATER	6:00 PM

*Page is from Touch for Health Complete Edition

THE WHEEL

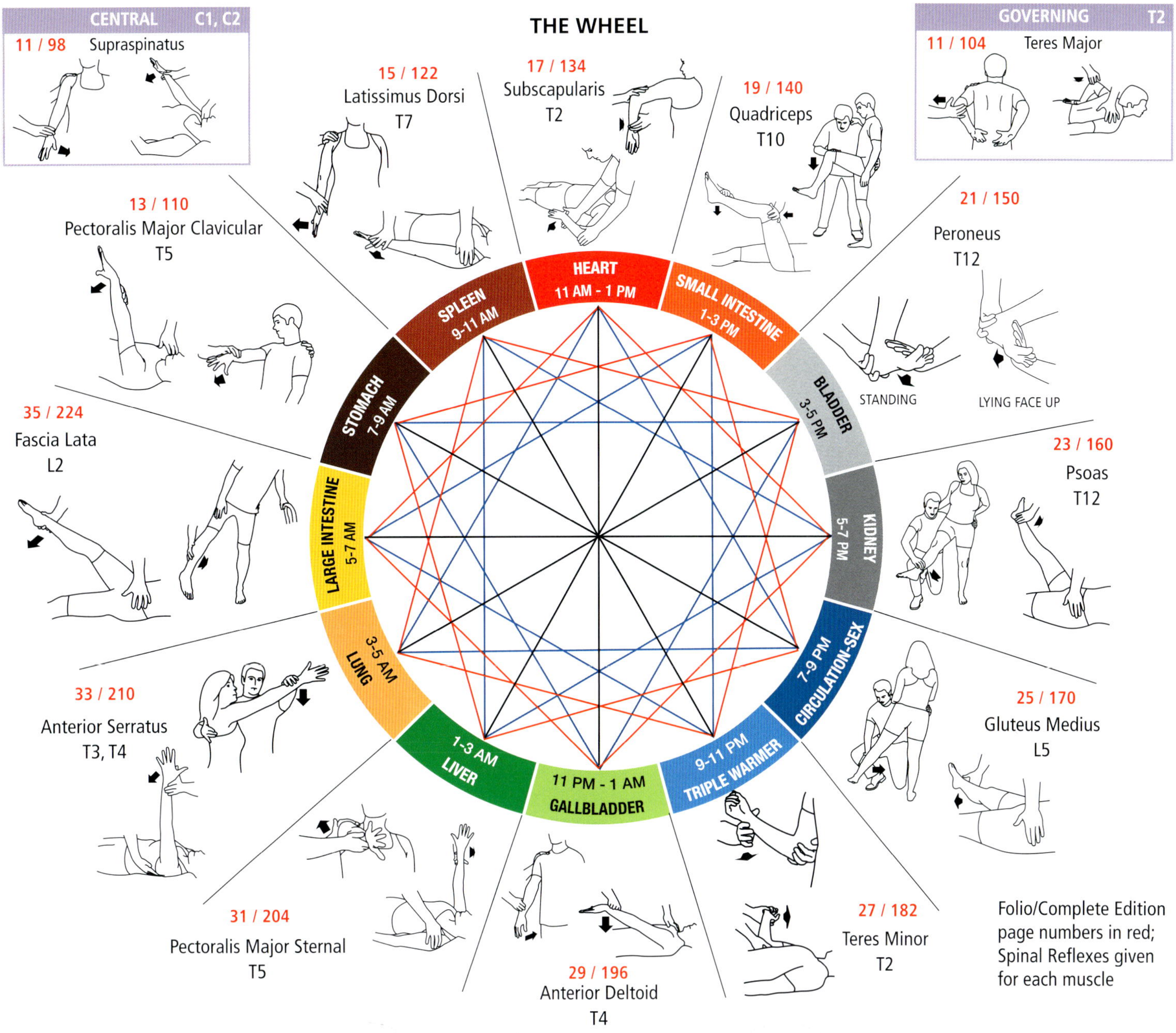

CENTRAL C1, C2
11 / 98 Supraspinatus

GOVERNING T2
11 / 104 Teres Major

15 / 122
Latissimus Dorsi
T7

17 / 134
Subscapularis
T2

19 / 140
Quadriceps
T10

13 / 110
Pectoralis Major Clavicular
T5

21 / 150
Peroneus
T12

STANDING

LYING FACE UP

35 / 224
Fascia Lata
L2

23 / 160
Psoas
T12

HEART
11 AM - 1 PM

SMALL INTESTINE
1-3 PM

BLADDER
3-5 PM

KIDNEY
5-7 PM

CIRCULATION-SEX
7-9 PM

TRIPLE WARMER
9-11 PM

GALLBLADDER
11 PM - 1 AM

LIVER
1-3 AM

LUNG
3-5 AM

LARGE INTESTINE
5-7 AM

STOMACH
7-9 AM

SPLEEN
9-11 AM

33 / 210
Anterior Serratus
T3, T4

25 / 170
Gluteus Medius
L5

31 / 204
Pectoralis Major Sternal
T5

29 / 196
Anterior Deltoid
T4

27 / 182
Teres Minor
T2

Folio/Complete Edition page numbers in red; Spinal Reflexes given for each muscle

ALARM POINTS

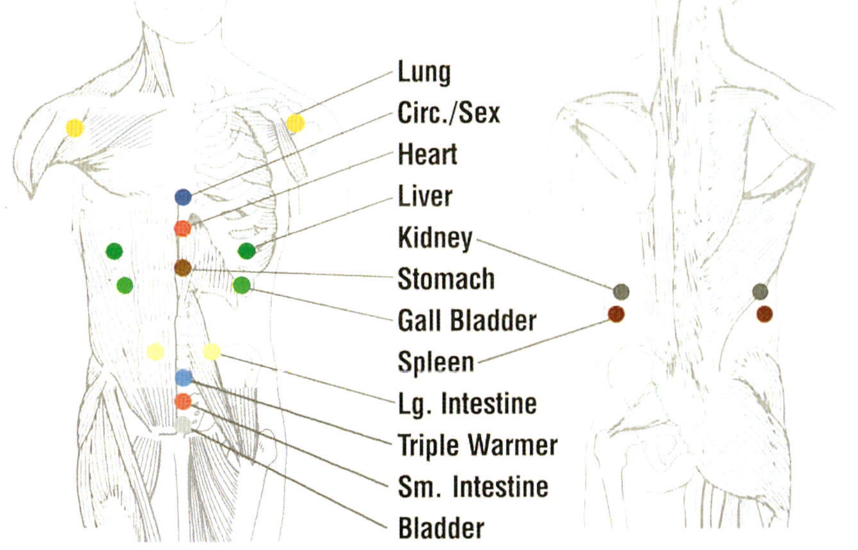

Lung
Circ./Sex
Heart
Liver
Kidney
Stomach
Gall Bladder
Spleen
Lg. Intestine
Triple Warmer
Sm. Intestine
Bladder

Circuit Locate with light touch and check indicator muscle for over-energy.

24 HOUR LAW

BALANCING THE MUSCLES, POSTURE & ENERGY "AS YOU GO"

In Touch for Health we use a *"Self-Responsibility"* model. **Always ask for permission** to touch, and check if there is any injury or other issue to avoid. If either partner wishes, they may say **"Stop" at any time**. Zip up your central meridian, switch-on, and drink some water. (See TFH Complete Edition for more details). Ideally, set up a **positive goal**/ intention/ or affirmation for the balance, check an Indicator Muscle for stress, and check at least one muscle (on right and left sides of the body) from each Meridian Reference Page. Or simply select an individual muscle based on where there is pain, dysfunction, etc. (See Muscle Map on back cover) If the same muscle is weak on both sides, gently stretch the skin up and down over the Spinal Reflex (SR). If weak on one side, firmly massage the Neurolymphatic Points (NL), retest and ***Challenge***. If more is needed, move on to lightly hold the Neurovasculars (NV), retest and Challenge. If more is needed, move on to tracing the Meridian, and continue with Muscle Origin/Insertion (O/I) points, Spindle Cells, Golgi Tendon and finally, the Acupressure Holding Points (AHP), as needed. After balancing the particular muscle, or all the muscles in sequence, reassess how you are feeling, and re-check your goal statement. If there is still stress, use Emotional Stress Release (holding the NV points for Pectoralis Major Clavicular/ Stomach Meridian). You can also circuit-locate each of the Reflex points (SR, NL, NV, Meridian end points, etc.) and see if the muscle switches on while holding the point. This indicates ahead of time which reflex will switch the muscle on. Work the reflex and challenge as usual. If NO reflex seems to switch the muscle on, check the Alarm Point (see below) for over-energy. If there is over-energy, hold the acupressure holding points ***to sedate***.

Challenging the Balancing Reflex

After switching a muscle on with a particular reflex, we may get additional benefit working more reflexes. Challenge the reflex by touching the point you just worked, and rechecking the muscle. If the muscle gets ***stronger,*** *work the same reflex* some more. If there is **no change** in the muscle response, *move on* to the next muscle. If the muscle gets ***weaker*** when challenging the reflex, move on to the *next reflex*. In the case of SR, if both sides switch on, move on. If one side is still weak, move on to the NL points, and then challenge the NL as above.

....

ASSESSMENT OR 1-POINT BALANCING

According to the 24-Hour Wheel & The Five Elements

Instead of balancing "as you go", just test all of the muscles first and look for a pattern based on the 24-hr Wheel or Five Elements. The key point may correct all of the imbalances in the system with one energy reflex. Contemplating the Metaphors related to such a key point often yields surprising insights... AND BALANCES THE MUSCLES AND ENERGY!

Muscles that unlock or feel weak are "unbalanced", either because of too much or too little energy. Circuit-locate the **Alarm Points** using a light touch to indicate which are over-energy (Pulse Points also indicate over-energy in the related meridians). If the IM changes while circuit-locating the related Alarm Point, it is considered over-energy, whether the related muscle is switched off or not. If the muscle is switched off (tests weak), and the Alarm Point does not indicate over-energy, then it must be under-energy.

Patterns Illustrated on the Wheel Diagram:

- **Beaver Dam**
  When there is an over-energy meridian, followed in a *clockwise* direction by two or more under-energy muscles, Work the reflexes of the first under-energy muscle following the over-energy.

THE 5-ELEMENTS, EMOTIONS AND SOUNDS

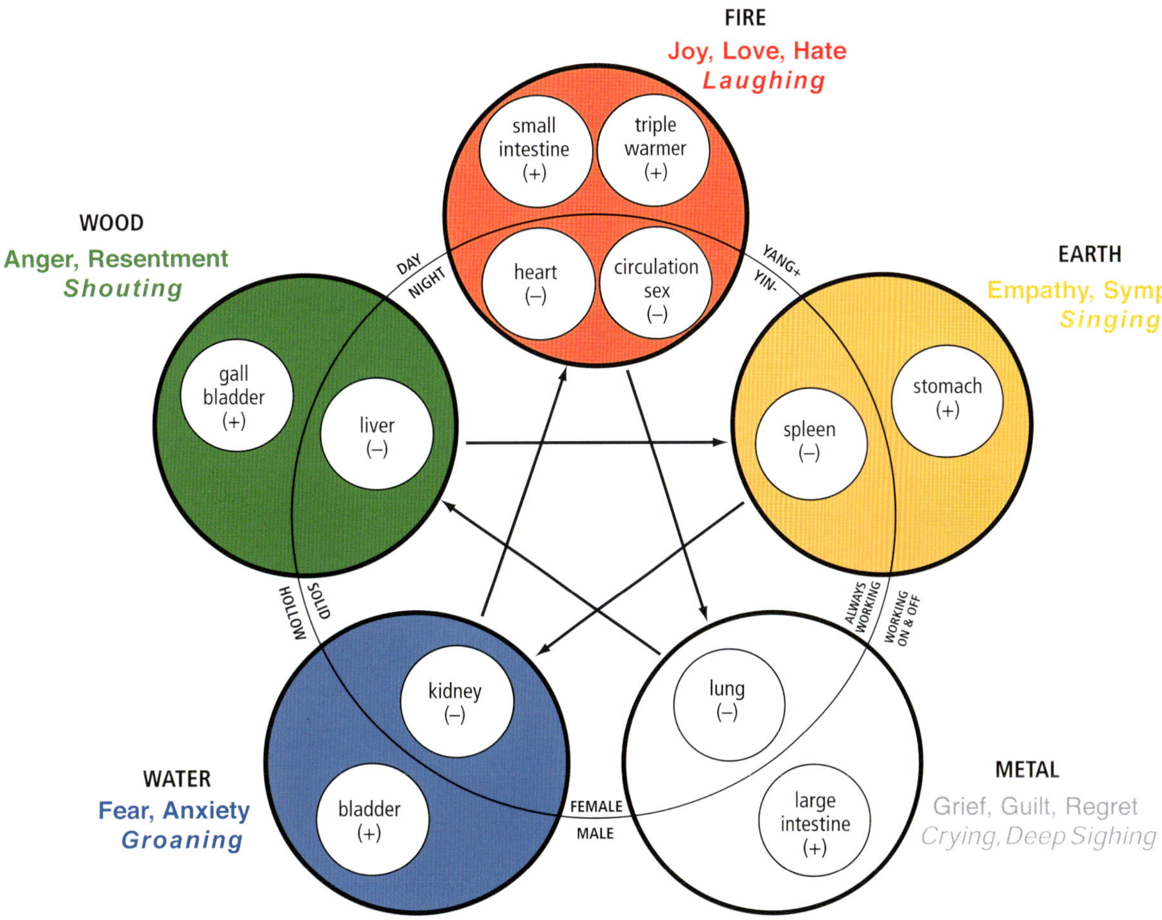

FIRE
Joy, Love, Hate
Laughing

small intestine (+), triple warmer (+), heart (–), circulation sex (–)

EARTH
Empathy, Sympathy
Singing

spleen (–), stomach (+)

METAL
Grief, Guilt, Regret
Crying, Deep Sighing

lung (–), large intestine (+)

WATER
Fear, Anxiety
Groaning

kidney (–), bladder (+)

WOOD
Anger, Resentment
Shouting

gall bladder (+), liver (–)

DAY / NIGHT
YANG+ / YIN-
ALWAYS WORKING / WORKING ON & OFF
FEMALE / MALE
SOLID / HOLLOW

METAPHOR WHEEL

	WOOD	FIRE	EARTH	METAL	WATER
ELEMENT	WOOD	FIRE	EARTH	METAL	WATER
SEASON	spring	summer	late summer	autumn	winter
CLIMATE	wind	heat	humidity	dryness	cold
ODOR	rancid	scorched	fragrant	rotten	putrid
TASTE	sour	bitter	sweet	pungent	salty
EMOTION	anger	joy	sympathy	grief	fear
SOUND	shouting	laughing	singing	weeping	groaning
FORTIFIES	ligaments	arteries	muscles	skin & hair	bones
POWER	birth	mature	decrease	balance	emphasize
FAITH WORLDVIEW	intuitive/projective	literal/mythic	conventional	responsible	universal

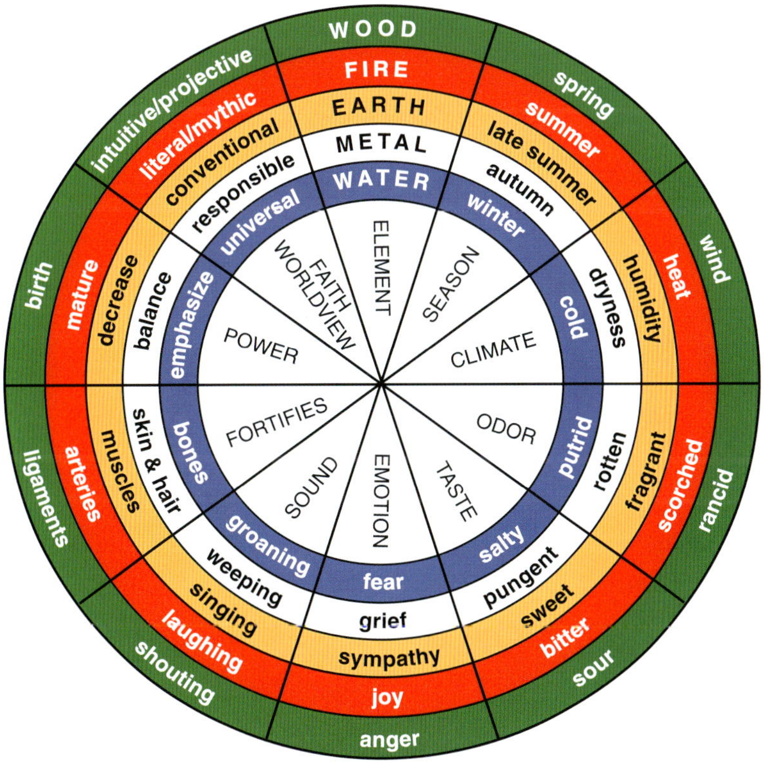

PULSE CHECK

LEFT HAND

LIGHT TOUCH
- Small Intestine
- Gallbladder
- Bladder

DEEP TOUCH
- Heart
- Liver
- Kidney

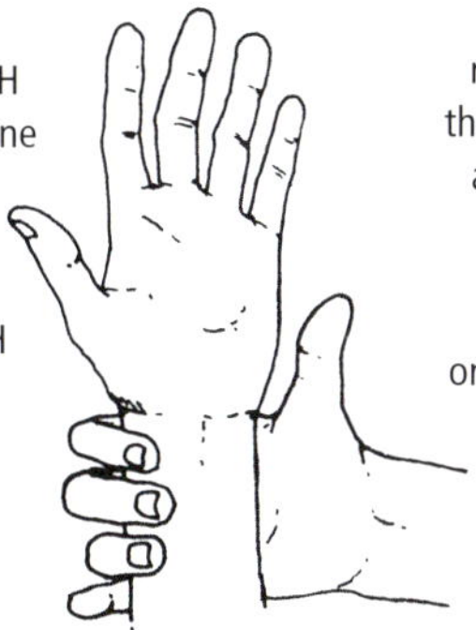

RIGHT HAND

LIGHT TOUCH
- Large Intestine
- Stomach
- Triple Warmer

DEEP TOUCH
- Lung
- Spleen
- Circulation-Sex

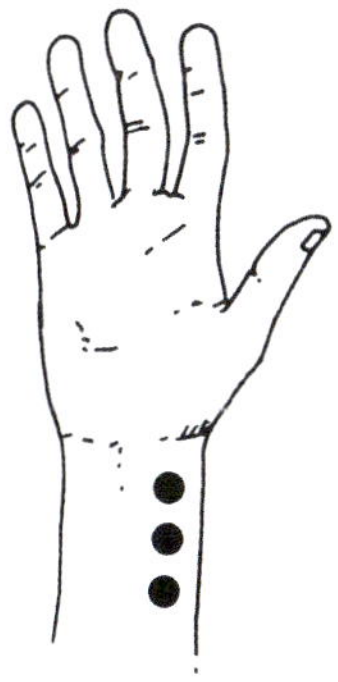

Use a light touch to represent the energy of the three Yang meridians and deep touch for Yin.

Using the Quadriceps or another leg muscle as an indicator muscle, note if there is a change while lightly holding the three fingers on the wrist. If there is, then check each finger separately to determine which Yang meridians have over-energy.

Using deep pressure, repeat with three fingers, which represent the Yin meridians. Then go to the opposite wrist and test in the same way.

- **Midday / Midnight Relationship**
  ***Black* "Spokes"** on the wheel show pairs of meridians whose ebb and flow are opposite each other on the clock. If one is over-energy, and the other is under-energy, work the reflexes of the muscle related to the under-energy.

- **Triangles and Squares**
  If there are 2 under-energy and 1 over-energy meridian on a ***Blue* Triangle** (3 meridians running same part of the body), Work the reflexes of the first under-energy muscle following the over-energy clockwise on the *triangle*. Similarly, If there are 3 under-energy and 1 over-energy meridian on a ***Red* Square** (4 meridians run a complete circuit of the body) work the reflexes of the first under-energy muscle following the over-energy clockwise on the *square*.

Patterns Illustrated on the Five-Elements Diagram:

The Five-Elements Diagram illustrates the **Shen** (or Creation) Cycle and the **Ko** (or Control) Cycle. Check the muscles and Alarm points to establish the pattern. Work the reflexes of the muscle related to the first under-energy ***YIN meridian*** (begin with Yin) following any over-energy in a clockwise direction. Follow either the Shen or Ko cycle.

Circuit Locate to Confirm the Key Point:

Circuit-locate the Neurolymphatic point of the muscle/meridian that looks like the key point while rechecking any *other* unlocking muscles. The other muscles should switch on while holding the NL point, confirming your key point will balance all the muscles/meridians. Work the reflexes of the key muscle, and recheck all muscles to confirm that they are now locked. Balance any remaining weak muscles individually.

....

TOUCH FOR HEALTH METAPHORS

In TFH we use muscle tests to get a sense of the energy flow in the meridians. We develop goals, assess the flow of energy, use various reflexes to balance energy and then reassess how we feel. Our purpose is to increase awareness of all of the aspects of our whole Soul and to facilitate the flow of energy and communication between all of the cells, organs and organ systems, between the conscious mind, the unconscious, our intuition, and our connection to Chi, life energy, or God. We can contemplate the metaphors associated with the Five Element Metaphors, Organ Functions, and Muscle Functions/Motions to get a more holistic sense of what is happening in our life. Consider each Metaphor as a symbol for some aspect of your life and see what it suggests to you. The questions provided here are merely examples. Consider your own ideas and intuition to be the highest authority for YOU.

The Central and Governing Meridians represent the major **Yin and Yang polarities**, and act as the central **"storage battery".** The Creative/ Nurturing (Sheng) Functions and the Controlling/Destructive (Ko) functions of the **entire Meridian System are working together here**. They relate to ALL Meridians and Elements globally, as a SYSTEM.

CENTRAL MERIDIAN (CONCEPTION VESSEL)

MAJOR YIN, *SHENG CYCLE*, RECEIVING, CONCEIVING, BRAIN

What subtle, small thing or idea do you need to release to reach your goal?
Or, do you need to receive or accept something?
How is your brain functioning?
Are you using your intelligence AND wisdom?

Color (**Violet/shadow:)** What might the color violet mean? (creative aspect of shadow, darkness, night, black & white)

Season (nurturing aspects of seasons:) Does the cycle of changing seasons nurture you or not?

Climate (**All beneficial climate:)** Is the climate and atmosphere enriching your life?

Odor (**Nurturing through smell:)** How does aroma nurture you? Do you nurture appreciation of smell?

Taste (**Creative aspects of taste:)** Are flavors and experiences nurturing your creativity and vitality?

Emotion (**Nurturing emotion:)** Do your emotions flow and enrich your life or are they blocked or toxic?

Sound (**Nurturing sound:)** Does sound enrich your life or are you sensitive to noise, easily annoyed?

Fortifies/Body Parts (integrated whole body:) How is the structure, posture and attitude of your interrelated body parts? Does your body support and enrich your life?

(Personal) Power(**Creative & procreative powers:)** Do the changes of season and stages of your life allow you new ways to fulfill your purposes? Do you find inspiration in changes in life and personal evolution?

Faith/Worldview (**Creative and nurturing aspects of belief:)** Do your beliefs and thinking processes support your vitality and creativity?

The **MUSCLE** related to Central Meridian is **Supraspinatus:** What subtle, small, yet Powerful action or initiative do you need to begin? Let go? Accept? Are you a "night person" or a "morning person"?

GOVERNING MERIDIAN/VESSEL

MAJOR YANG, *KO CYCLE*, ACTION, CONTROLLING, DESTRUCTION, SPINE

How do you feel about nighttime vs. daytime?
How is your life structured and controlled, too much or too little?
Is your life as a whole destructive, well-structured, too controlled, too chaotic or over-active?

Color (Violet/Sunlight): What might violet mean? (white light (sunlight), daytime, full spectrum color)

Season (Control/Destructive aspects of seasons): How does the cycle of changing seasons control your life and your decisions? What is destructive, or needs to be discarded with the changing of seasons?

Climate (Structural/harmful aspects of climate): Is the climate and atmosphere dictating your life? Is there something harmful, limiting, or constructive to you in your general environment or climate?

Odor (Controlling/destructive aspects of smell): How do smells affect you? Are they overwhelming to you or do they serve a valuable purpose? Do you "follow your nose"? Ruled by emotions or moods?

Taste (Controlling/destructive aspects of taste): Are you controlled by your tastes, or are you able to balance your desires and cravings with your wisdom and intelligent choices? Do you have a taste for any foods or activities that are destructive to you or others?

Emotion (Controlling/destructive aspects of emotion): Do your emotions flow and enrich your life or are they blocked or toxic? Are you (too much) in control of your emotions, or are you controlled, at the mercy of, or overwhelmed by your emotions?

Sound (Controlling/destructive aspects of sound): Are you able to structure and manage the sounds and music of your life, or is there discord, harmful words or sounds in your life? (Over) sensitive to sound?

Fortifies/body parts **(Controlling/destructive aspects of the body):** How is the overall structure and interrelation of all of your body parts? Does your body support and enrich your life, or are your purposes thwarted by the shape and function of your body?

(Personal) Power(Controlling and destructive powers): Are you able to stay organized and keep structure in your life with changing circumstances, seasons and stages of your life? Is your personal evolution hampered by circumstances? Are you appropriately exerting control and even your destructive powers?

Faith/Worldview (Controlling/destructive aspects of belief): Do your beliefs and thinking processes create a foundation and structure for ethical and productive behavior or does your perception of the world lead to disorganization, struggle, or destructive behavior? Are you aware of your beliefs, or unsure of reality?

The **MUSCLE** related to Governing Meridian is **Teres Major:** What burden, weight, or obligation are you carrying? Is someone "twisting your arm behind your back?

CENTRAL: NIGHTTIME

RNA

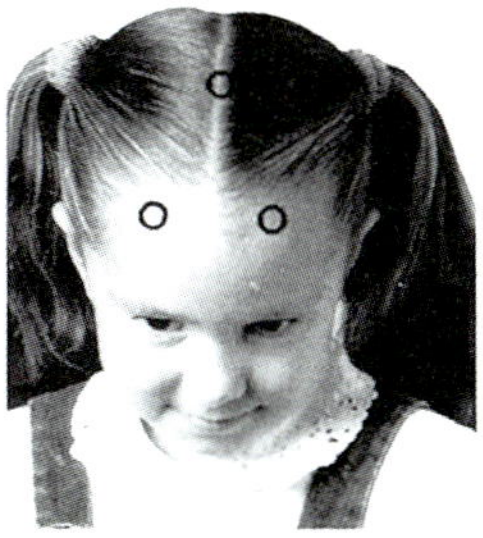

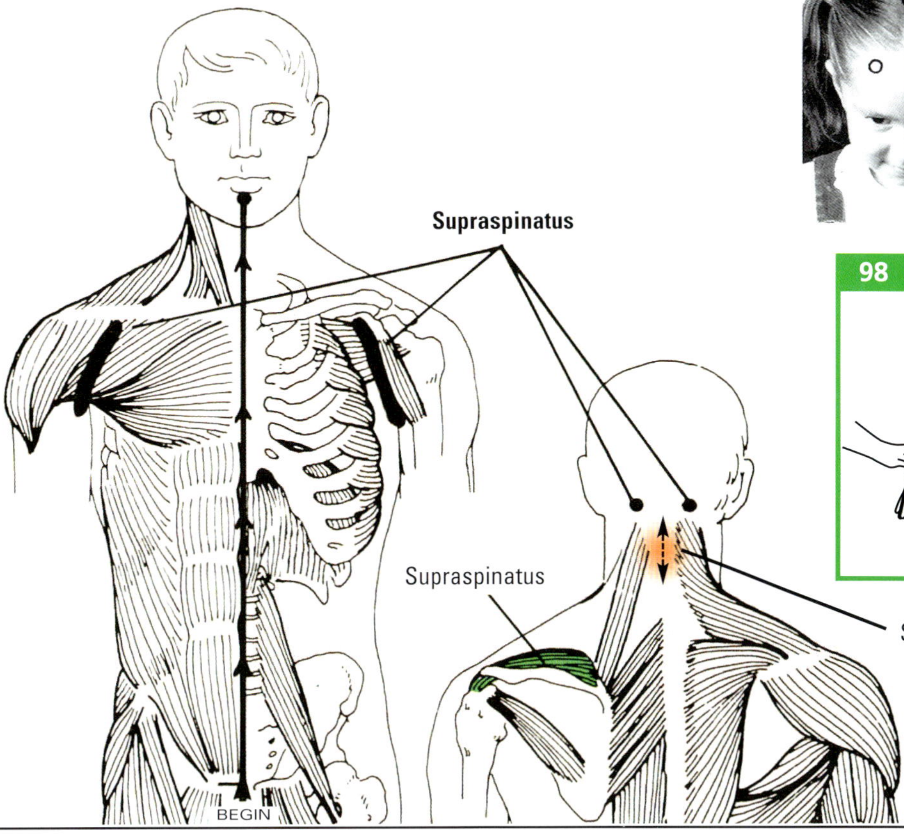

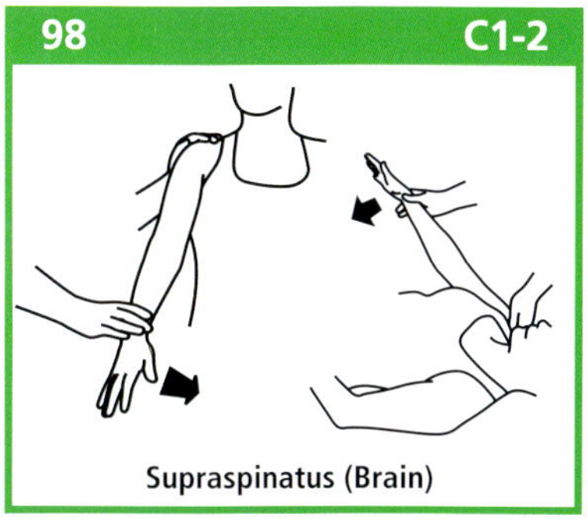

Supraspinatus (Brain)

GOVERNING: DAYTIME

Whole Protein

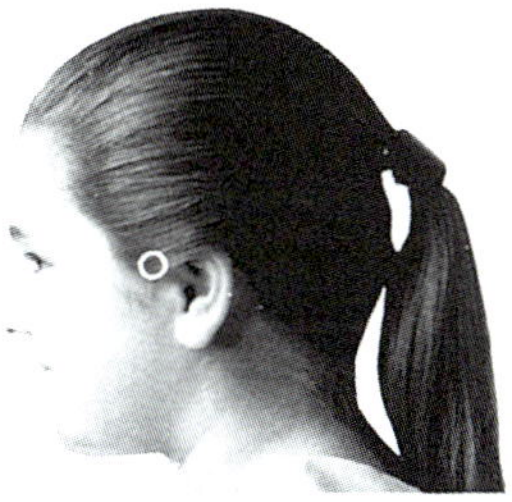

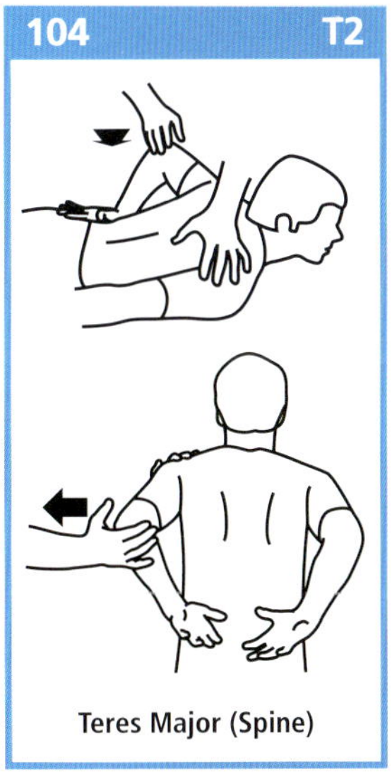

Teres Major (Spine)

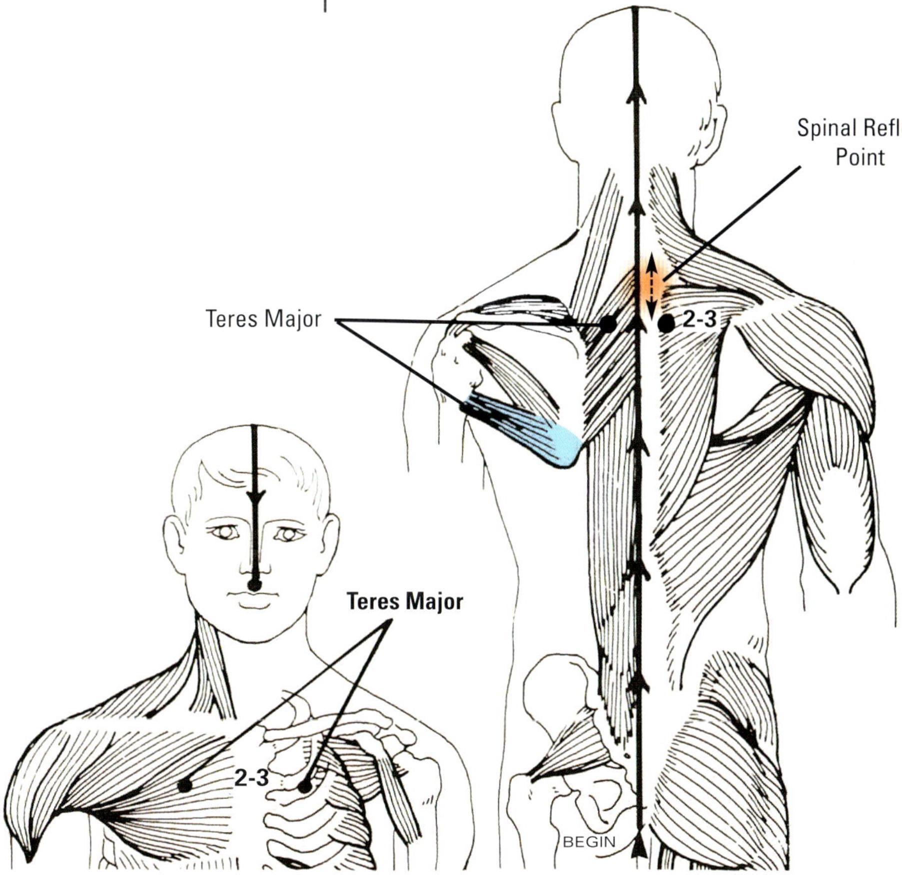

THE EARTH ELEMENT

CENTER, TRANSITION, STABILITY AND DYNAMIC CHANGE, THE LAND, THE SOIL, HOME

Do you have your feet on the ground or do you need to be grounded, rooted, stable? Can you handle Change, transition smoothly?

Color: **Yellow** What might the color yellow represent? Are you yellow or courageous?

Season: **Late Summer** Is it time for the harvest, or do you need to let things develop a little longer?

Climate: **Dampness/Humidity** Is fog hampering your progress or do you need *more* steam?

Odor: **Fragrant** Do you need to "smell the flowers" or focus on the effort to bring in the harvest?

Taste: **Sweet** What tastes Sweet in your life/goals? Is something too sweet or "saccharin"?

Emotion: **Sympathy/Empathy** Do you need empathy/sympathy or to relate to others' feelings?

Sound: **Singing** Do you need enthusiasm, expression, singing, or do you "sing" or tell too much?

Fortifies: **Muscles** Do you need more power/movement or do you need stillness and patience?

Personal Power: **Decrease** What can you decrease to allow you more (Personal) Power in your life?

Faith/Worldview: Late Adolescence or **Conventional/Synthetic Faith**
What are your values vs. the values of your peer group, community or culture?

STOMACH MERIDIAN FUNCTION	**7-9 AM**

Are you receiving the proper resources to fulfill your purposes? Are you able to use your resources efficiently? What nutrient, emotion, or idea are you digesting? What is difficult for to swallow or gives you a stomachache (physical, emotional, etc) or inhibits free breathing, figuratively or literally?

PECTORALIS MAJOR CLAVICULAR: Do you need to hold your chest up or are you too proud?

LEVATOR SCAPULAE: Are you keeping your head on straight/ your nose up, literally or figuratively?

NECK MUSCLES:

- **Anterior Neck flexors:** Are you having trouble holding your head up, literally or figuratively?
- **Posterior Neck Extensors:** Are you literally sticking your neck out, or figuratively taking risks/chances?

BRACHIORADIALIS: Can you physically reach behind you? Ignoring things in your blind spot?

 |

STOMACH: 7-9 AM

Neck Flexors & Extensors: Niacin, B6, G Iodine
Pectoralis Major Clavicular: B, G, HCl
Levator Scapulae: B
Brachiordialis: B

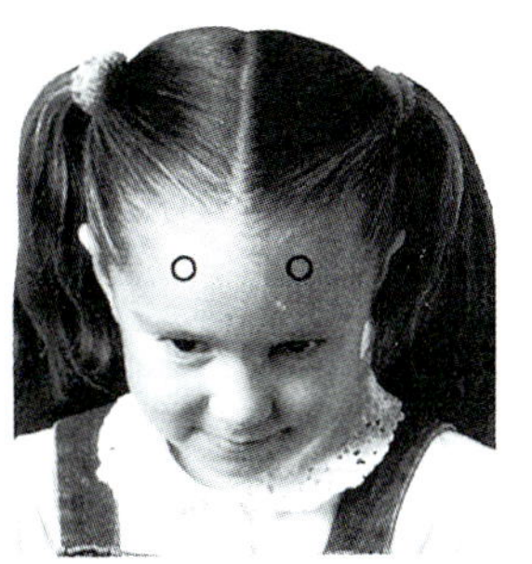

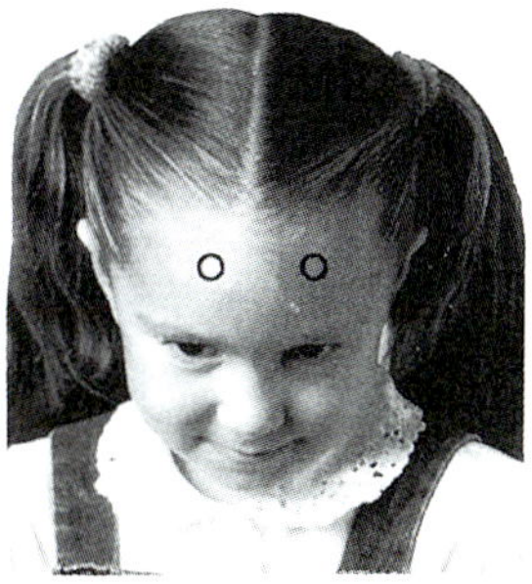

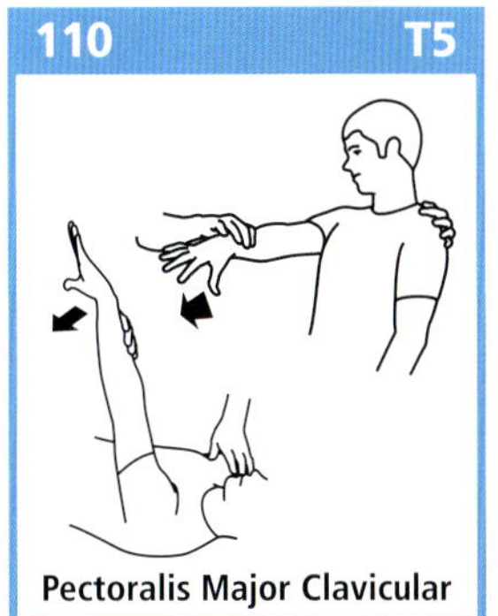
110 T5

Pectoralis Major Clavicular

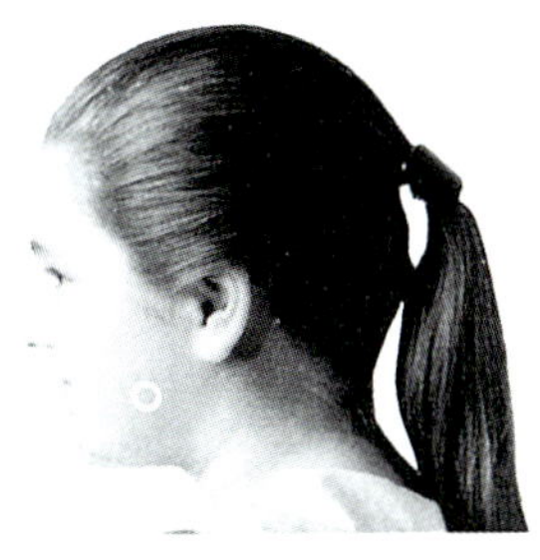

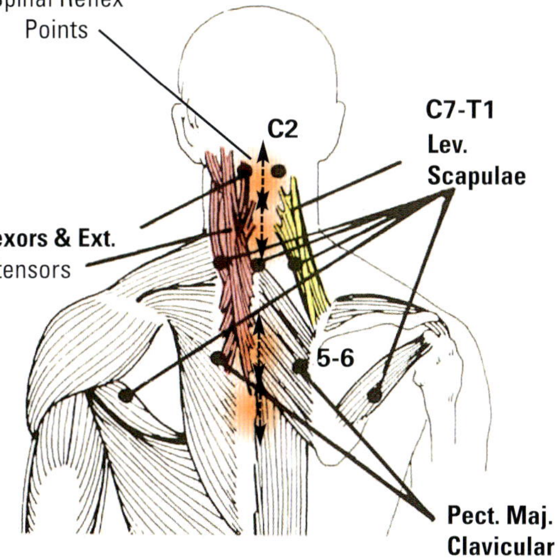

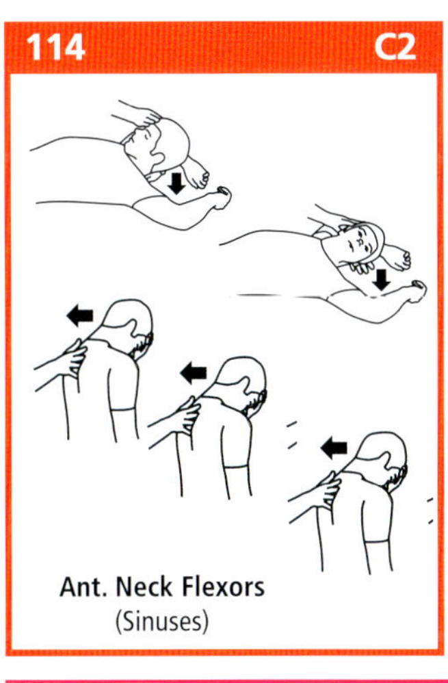
114 C2

Ant. Neck Flexors
(Sinuses)

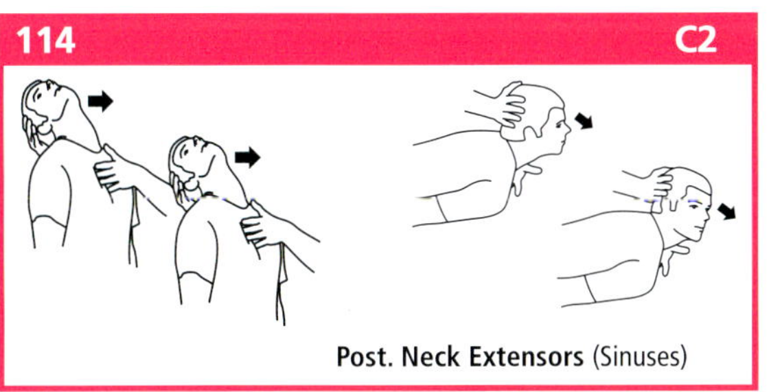
114 C2

Post. Neck Extensors (Sinuses)

BEGIN

Ant. Neck Flexors

Levator Scap.

Neck Flexors & Extensors

Pect. Maj. Clav.

5-6
Pect. Maj. Clav.
Brachioradialis
Left side only

Alarm Point

Brachioradialis

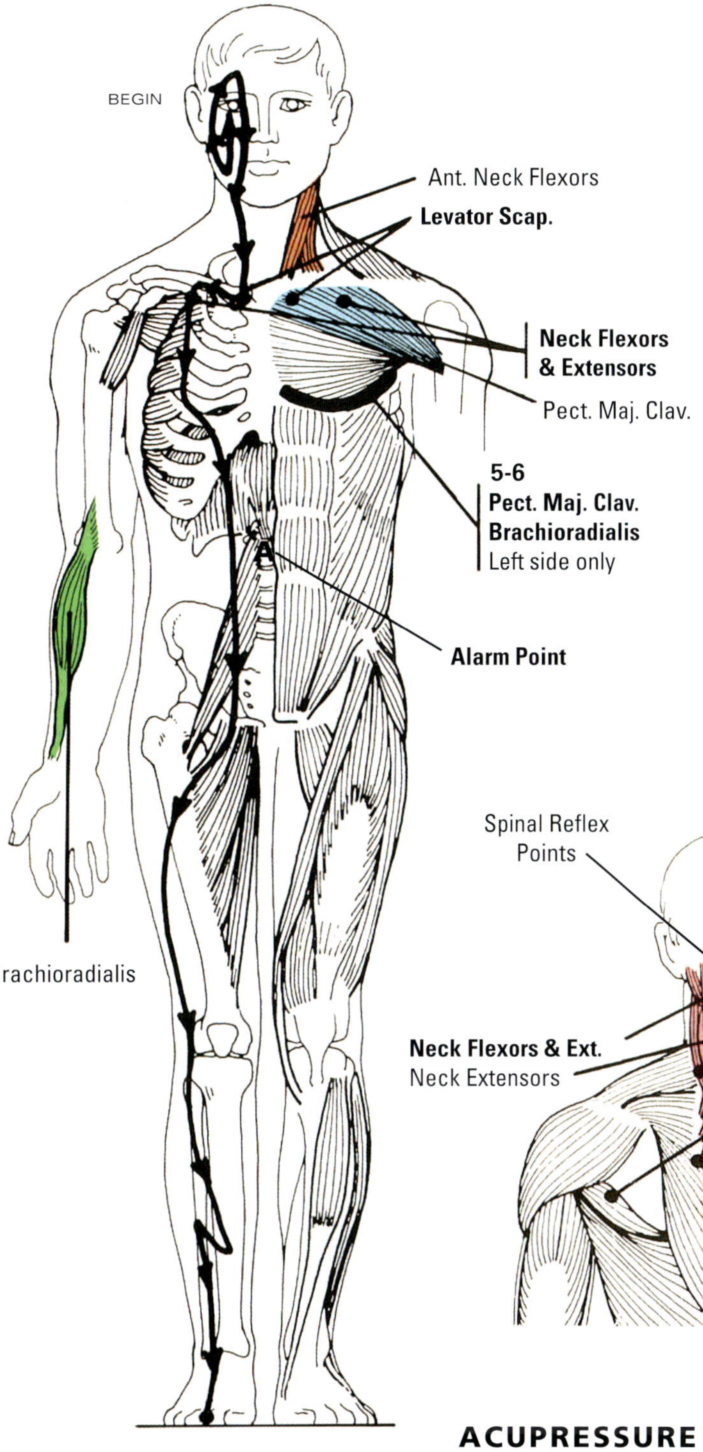

112 C5, T8

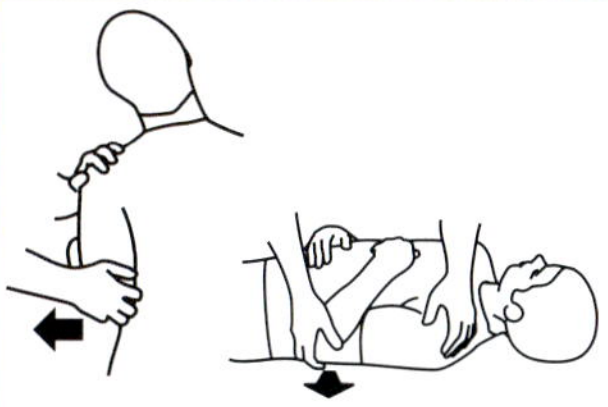

Levator Scapulae

116 T12

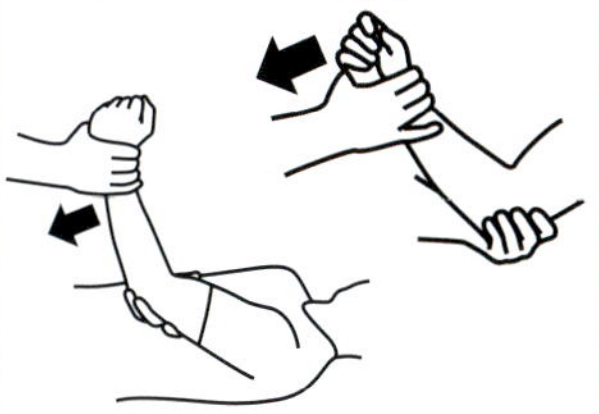

Brachioradialis

Spinal Reflex Points

C2

C7-T1
Lev. Scapulae

Neck Flexors & Ext.
Neck Extensors

5-6

Pect. Maj. Clavicular

ACUPRESSURE HOLDING POINTS

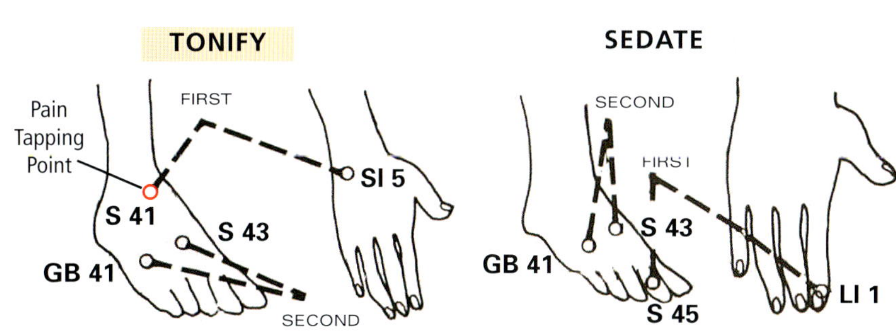

THE EARTH ELEMENT

CENTER, TRANSITION, STABILITY AND DYNAMIC CHANGE, THE LAND, THE SOIL, HOME

Do you have your feet on the ground or do you need to be grounded, rooted, stable? Can you handle Change, transition smoothly?

Color: **Yellow** What might the color yellow represent? Are you yellow or courageous?

Season: **Late Summer** Is it time for the harvest, or do you need to let things develop a little longer?

Climate: **Dampness/Humidity** Is fog hampering your progress or do you need *more* steam?

Odor: **Fragrant** Do you need to "smell the flowers" or focus on the effort to bring in the harvest?

Taste: **Sweet** What tastes Sweet in your life/goals? Is something too sweet or "saccharin"?

Emotion: **Sympathy/Empathy** Do you need empathy/ sympathy to relate to others' feelings?

Sound: **Singing** Do you need enthusiasm, expression, singing, or do you "sing" or tell too much?

Fortifies: **Muscles** Do you need more power/movement or do you need stillness and patience?

Personal Power: **Decrease** What can you decrease to allow you more (Personal) Power in your life?

Faith/Worldview: Late Adolescence or **Conventional/Synthetic Faith**
What are your values vs. the values of your peer group, community or culture?

SPLEEN MERIDIAN FUNCTION	9-11 AM

Are you burdened with toxic dietary, mental, chemical, spiritual materials? Are you breaking down problems into digestible parts?

LATISSIMUS DORSI: Are you taking swings, striking at things, inhibited from making large gestures?

MIDDLE TRAPEZIUS: Are you attempting to embrace too much? Need to open your arms wide?

LOWER TRAPEZIUS: Are you too open, vulnerable, or do you need to embrace the whole sky?

OPPONENS POLLICIS LONGUS: What do you need to get a grip on? Are you holding on too tightly?

TRICEPS: Are you reaching out/gathering in enough or not enough, literally or figuratively?

SPLEEN 9-11 AM

Latissimus Dorsi: A, F, HCl
Triceps: A
Opponens Pollicis Longus: B6, A
Middle Trapezius: C
Lower Trapezius: F, G, C

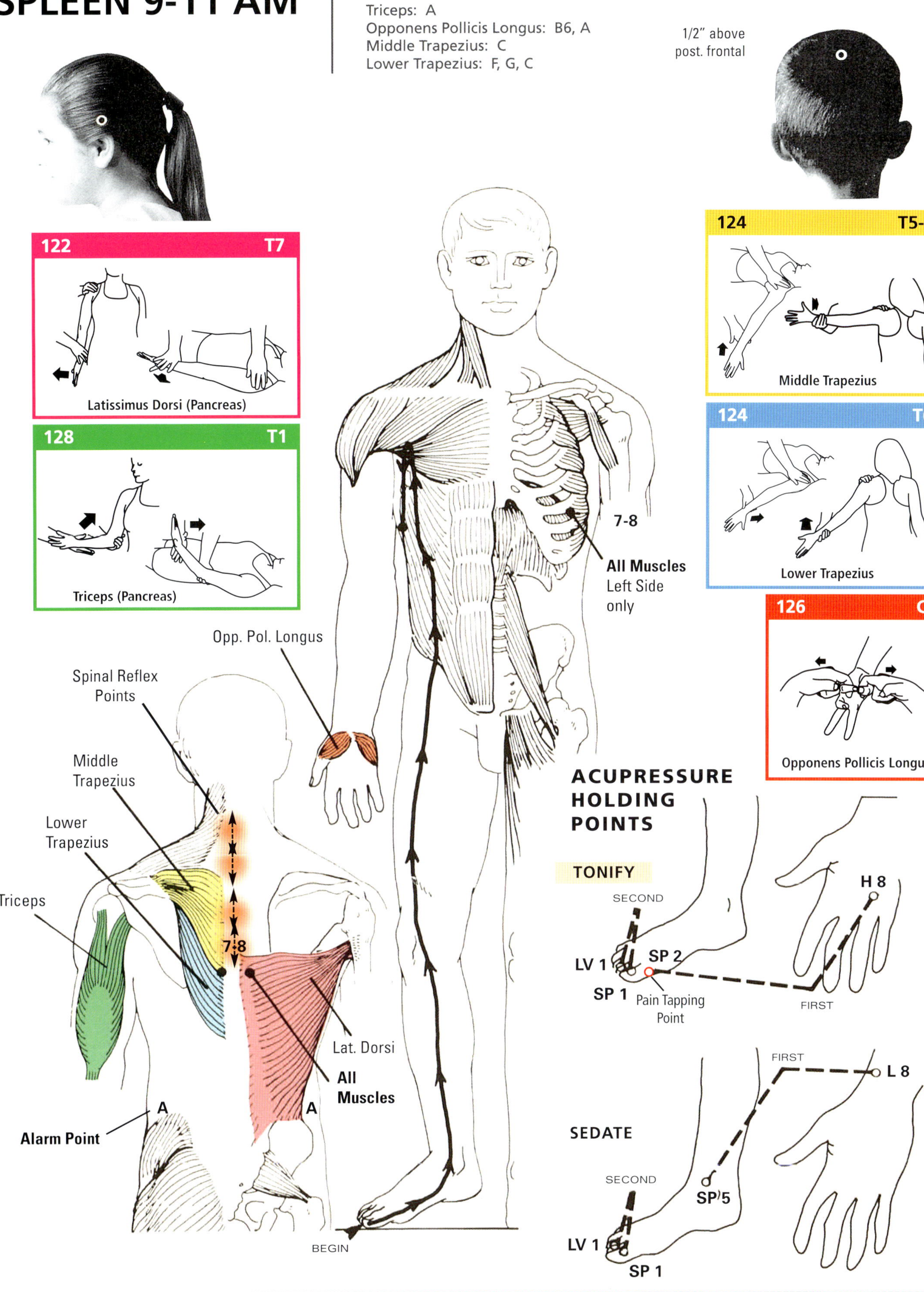

THE FIRE ELEMENT

Heat, Burning, Energy, Passion, Action, Stimulation, Challenges, Danger

Do you have "fire in the belly", passion and energy for life? Are you too passionate, burning up your energy stores, burning those around you, or are you too cold, and unable to be passionate?

Color:Red Do you have enough Red in your life, or too much Red? Red alert?

Season: Summer Do you have "fun in the sun", or are you sensitive to light, sapped of energy?

Climate: Heat Can you take the Heat, or is the stress and pressure overwhelming? Are you too passionate, playing it too cool, or getting burned out? Do you run Hot or Cold? Need excitement?

Odor: Scorched Are you scorched by the elements, traumatic experiences, the passions, demands, or criticisms of others? Do you take risks, even at the cost of getting scorched? Smell danger?

Taste: Bitter What are your regrets or grudges? What's poisoning you? Too much stimulation, or not?

Emotion: Joy Do you need more Love and Joy in your life? Masking pain with a manic attitude/ drugs?

Sound: Laughing Do you enjoy mirth and Laughter. Avoid experiencing emotions by "laughing them off"? Have you laughed at the wrong moment? Been made fun of, laughed at, scorned or ridiculed?

Fortifies: Arteries Do you have a steady flow and distribution of the fuels and supplies to maintain your mental, emotional, spiritual and physical vitality? Does some part get poor circulation and go cold?

(Personal) Power: Mature Are you at ease with your limitations? Do you make full use of your capacities? Are you capricious? Do you experience childlike wonder and joy in life?

Faith/Worldview: Childhood/"School Years" or **Literal/Mythic Faith** Do you have a narrow, literal interpretation of rules, morals or beliefs? Are you conscious of conventions? Are you "re-inventing the wheel", "going it alone"? Do you expect precise reciprocity from others? Playing "tit for tat"?

HEART MERIDIAN FUNCTION	**11 AM-1 PM**

Do you have fluid circulation and communication within your Soul, or in your daily activities, literally or figuratively? Is there any conflict between your logical thinking, intuition, wisdom or emotional feelings? Is your heart in the right place? Are you physically fit?

SUBSCAPULARIS: What are you hiding or keeping private? What do you need to reveal? What do you feel in your heart as opposed to your head? Is someone twisting your arm? Any mysterious pains?

 |

HEART 11 AM-1 PM | G, E, B, Calcium

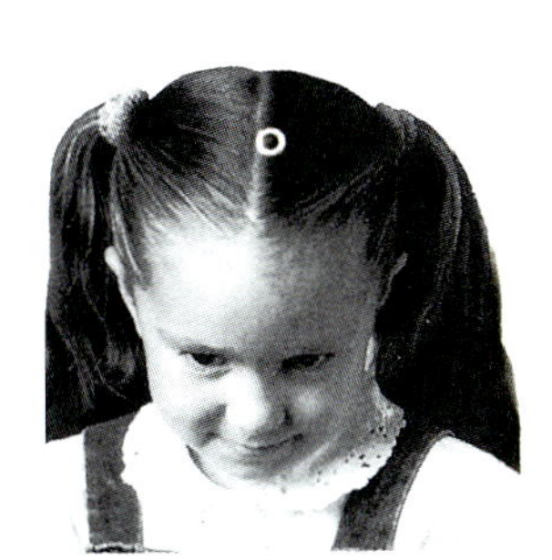

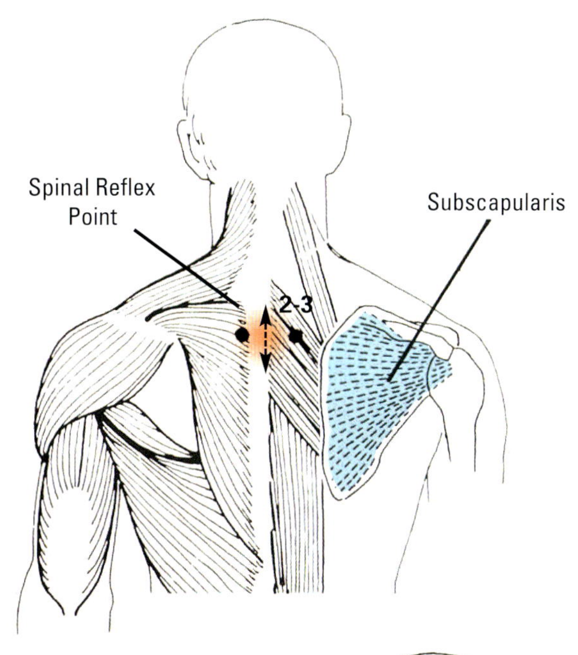

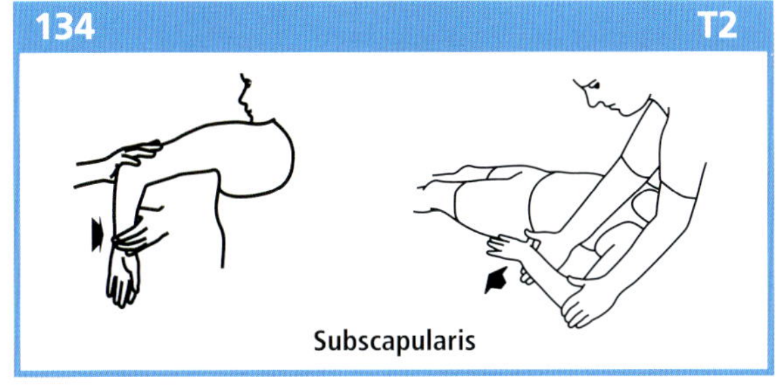

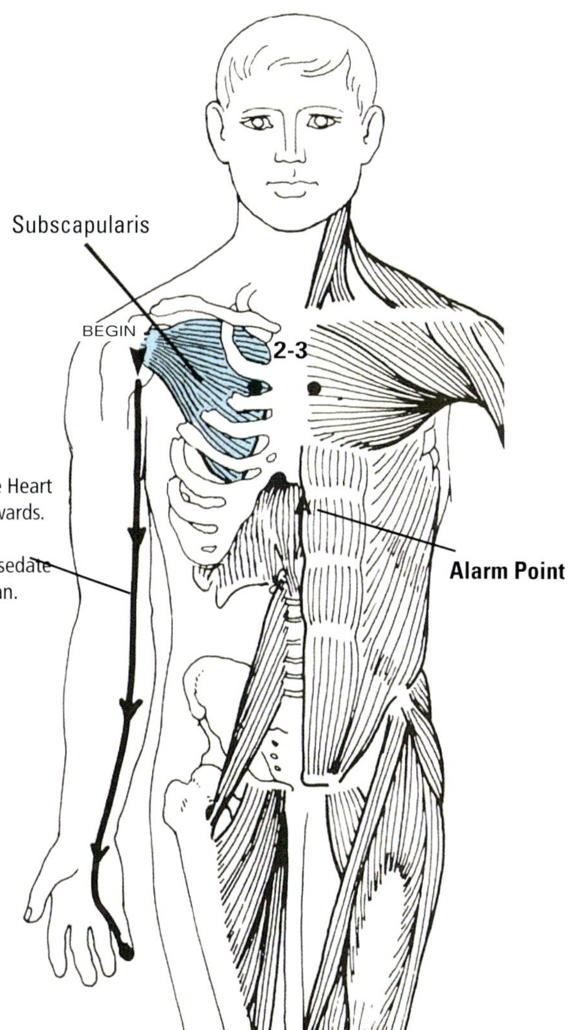

ACUPRESSURE HOLDING POINTS

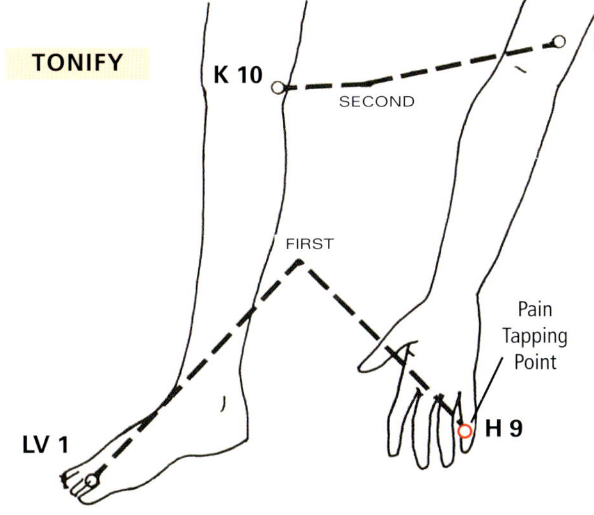

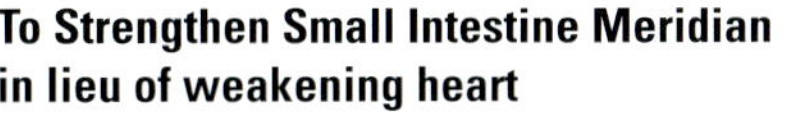

To Strengthen Small Intestine Meridian in lieu of weakening heart

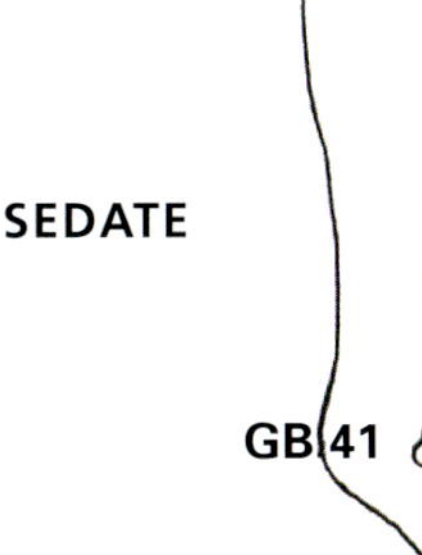

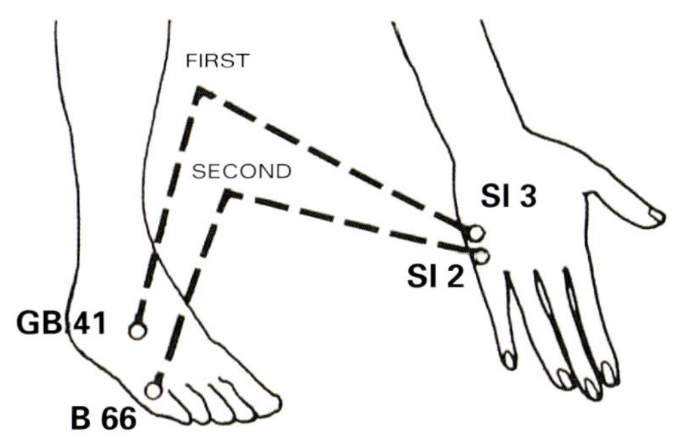

THE FIRE ELEMENT

Heat, Burning, Energy, Passion, Action, Stimulation, Challenges, Danger

Do you have "fire in the belly", passion and energy for life? Are you too passionate, burning up your energy stores, burning those around you, or are you too cold, and unable to be passionate?

Color:Red Do you have enough Red in your life, or too much Red? Red alert?

Season: Summer Do you have "fun in the sun", or are you sensitive to light, sapped of energy?

Climate: Heat Can you take the Heat, or is the stress and pressure overwhelming? Are you too passionate, playing it too cool, or getting burned out? Do you run Hot or Cold? Need excitement?

Odor: Scorched Are you scorched by the elements, traumatic experiences, the passions, demands, or criticisms of others? Do you take risks, even at the cost of getting scorched? Smell danger?

Taste: Bitter What are your regrets or grudges? What's poisoning you? Too much stimulation, or not?

Emotion: Joy Do you need more Love and Joy in your life? Masking pain with a manic attitude/ drugs?

Sound: Laughing Do you enjoy mirth and Laughter. Avoid experiencing emotions by "laughing them off"? Have you laughed at the wrong moment? Been made fun of, laughed at, scorned or ridiculed?

Fortifies: Arteries Do you have a steady flow and distribution of the fuels and supplies to maintain your mental, emotional, spiritual and physical vitality? Does some part get poor circulation and go cold?

(Personal) Power: Mature Are you at ease with your limitations? Do you make full use of your capacities? Are you capricious? Do you experience childlike wonder and joy in life?

Faith/Worldview: Childhood/"School Years" or **Literal/Mythic Faith** Do you have a narrow, literal interpretation of rules, morals or beliefs? Are you conscious of conventions? Are you "re-inventing the wheel", "going it alone"? Do you expect precise reciprocity from others? Playing "tit for tat"?

SMALL INTESTINE MERIDIAN FUNCTION | 1-3 PM

What is difficult to absorb, digest or gives you a stomach ache (physically, emotionally, etc) or inhibits free breathing, figuratively or literally?

QUADRICEPS: Stepping up or taking big steps? Climbing a mountain? Need to "put your foot down"?

ABDOMINALS: What is your posture/ attitude? Balanced, able to "make your moves?"

Off kilter?

 |

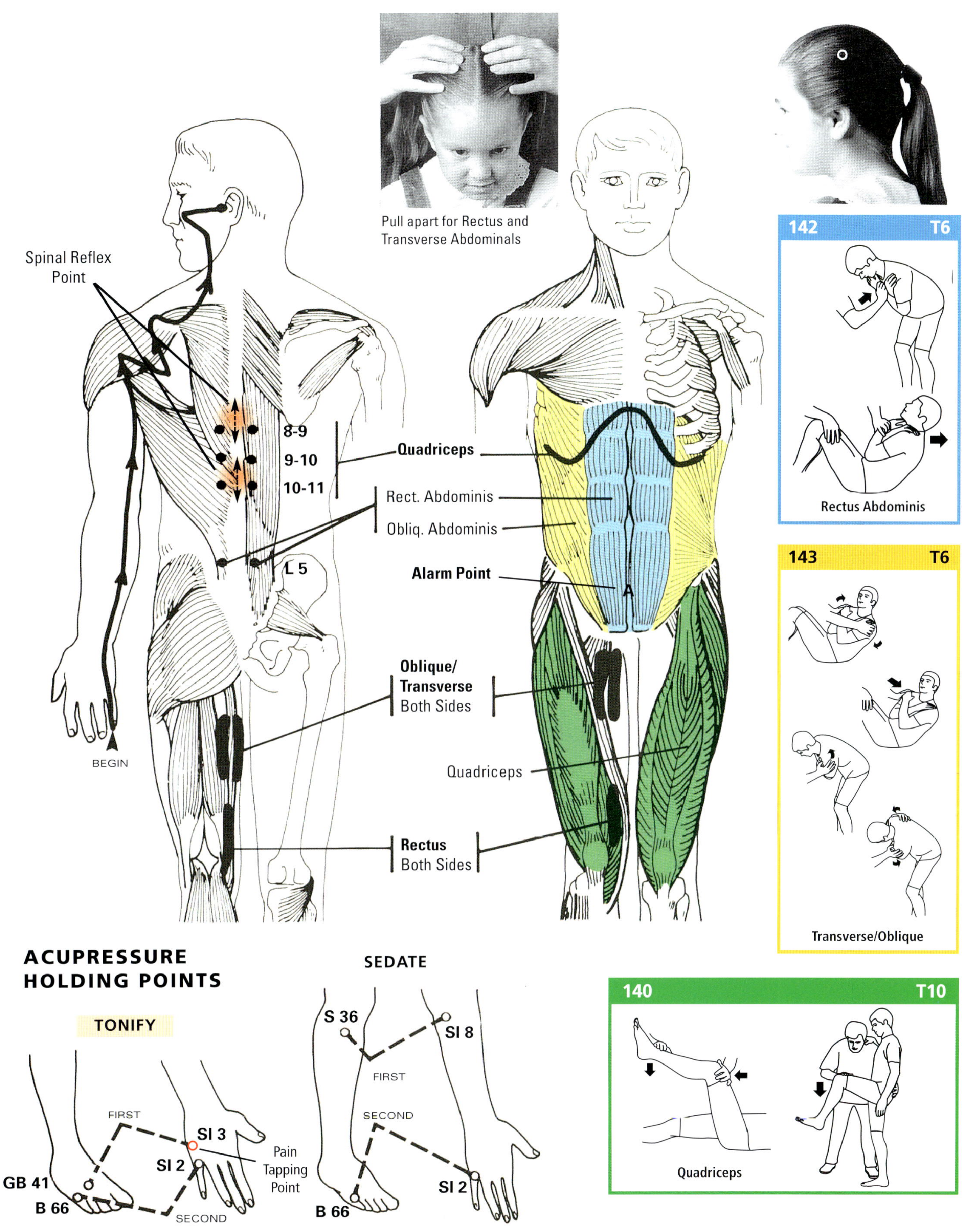
Pull apart for Rectus and Transverse Abdominals
Spinal Reflex Point
8-9
9-10
10-11
Quadriceps
Rect. Abdominis
Obliq. Abdominis
L 5
Alarm Point
A
BEGIN
Oblique/ Transverse Both Sides
Quadriceps
Rectus Both Sides
142
T6
Rectus Abdominis
143
T6
Transverse/Oblique
140
T10
Quadriceps
ACUPRESSURE HOLDING POINTS
TONIFY
FIRST
SI 3
SI 2
GB 41
B 66
SECOND
Pain Tapping Point
SEDATE
S 36
SI 8
FIRST
SECOND
B 66
SI 2

THE WATER ELEMENT

Fluidity/Flow, The Sea, Mystery, Sub/Un-consciousness, Purity, Abundance

Is there too much mystery, fear and risk, or do you need to overcome your fears and allow some uncertainty to fulfill your dreams?
How are things flowing, fast or slow?

Color: Blue What does blue mean to you in your life or in relation to your current goals? Are you blue?

Season: Winter Are you active when you need to contemplate or plan? Do you feel left out in the cold?

Climate: Cold Are you numbed by a harsh environment, or do you need to cool your passions?

Odor: Putrid What has died and needs to be buried? What is corrupt, offensive or disgusting?

Taste: Salty What needs to be preserved, "needs some salt" or must be "taken with a grain of salt"?

Emotion: Fear, Anxiety or **Awe** What are your Fears? Are you too worrisome or too fearless?

Sound: **Groaning** What do you need to Groan about, or are you groaning, or complaining too much?

Fortifies: Bones What do your Bones tell you? Can you be rigid or flexible? "skeletons in the closet"?

(Personal) Power: Emphasize What aspect of your life needs emphasis? What's neglected?

Faith/World View: Late Maturity/Death or **Reintegrative/Universalizing Faith**
Is it time to let go of concern for personal success, failure, contradiction, or injustice and simply concentrate on the greater good, or do you need be proactive in your own interests?

BLADDER MERIDIAN FUNCTION 3-5 PM

Are you hydrated, lubricated? Is energy and emotion freely flowing? What's too concentrated/ irritating? What do you need to release? What do you retain? Restrained?

PERONEUS: How are you mis-stepping? Should you watch your step or stop pussyfooting around?

SACROSPINALIS: What little things or big things are causing you tension, keeping you from standing straight?

ANTERIOR TIBIAL: Are you tapping your toes(in rhythm or impatience)? Do you need release?

POSTERIOR TIBIAL: Losing your balance? Are you kicking/being kicked? Are you running/ fighting?

BLADDER: 3-5 PM

Tibials: E, Calcium, Trace Minerals
Peroneus: B1, B, Calcium, Trace Minerals
Sacrospinalis: A, C

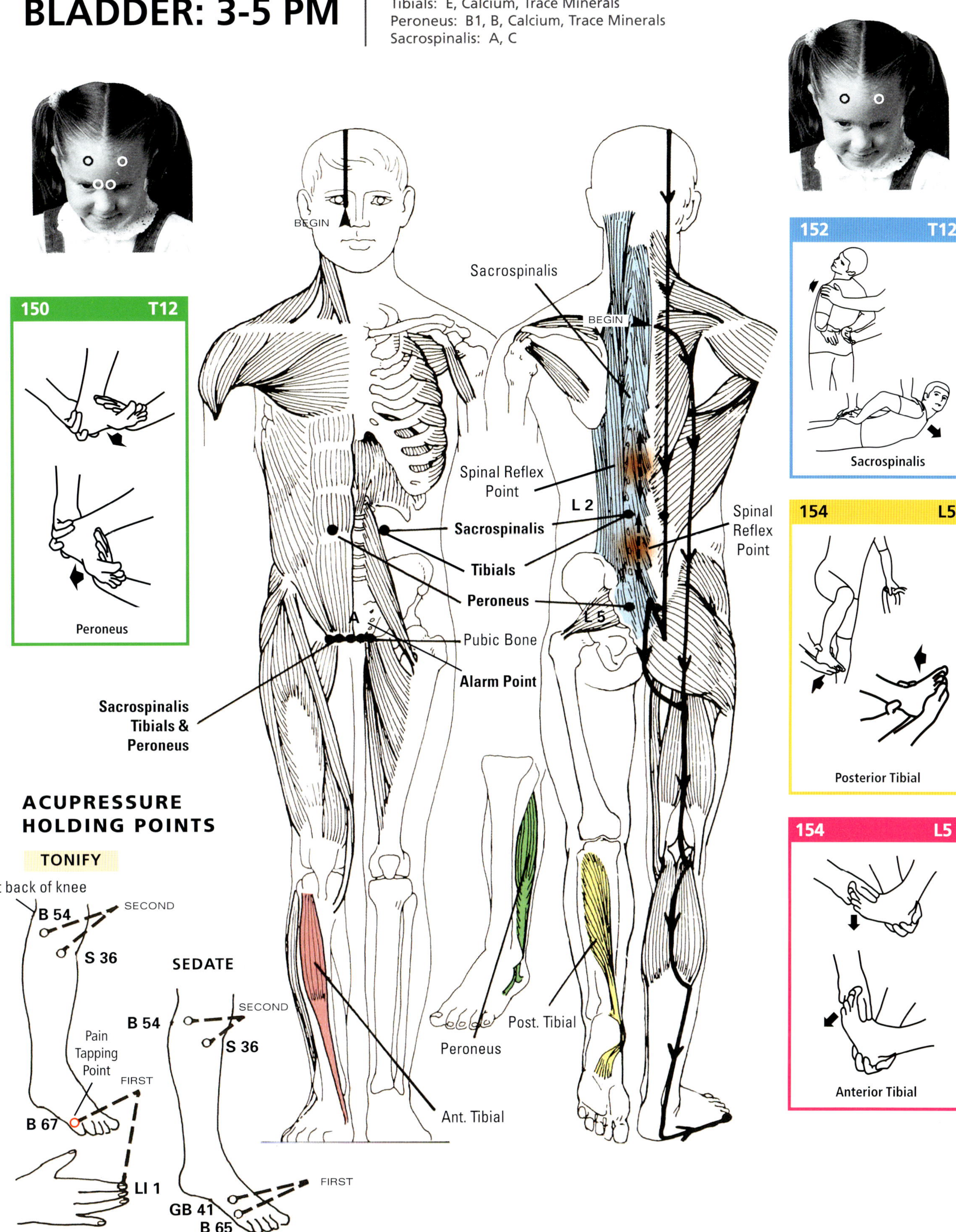

THE WATER ELEMENT

Fluidity/Flow, The Sea, Mystery, Sub/Un-consciousness, Purity, Abundance

**Is there too much mystery, fear and risk, or do you need to overcome your fears and allow some uncertainty to fulfill your dreams?
How are things flowing, fast or slow?**

Color: Blue What does blue mean to you in your life or in relation to your current goals? Are you blue?

Season: Winter Are you active when you need to contemplate or plan? Do you feel left out in the cold?

Climate: Cold Are you numbed by a harsh environment, or do you need to cool your passions?

Odor: Putrid What has died and needs to be buried? What is corrupt, offensive or disgusting?

Taste: Salty What needs to be preserved, "needs some salt" or must be "taken with a grain of salt"?

Emotion: Fear, Anxiety or **Awe** What are your Fears? Are you too worrisome or too fearless?

Sound: **Groaning** What do you need to Groan about, or are you groaning, or complaining too much?

Fortifies: Bones What do your Bones tell you? Can you be rigid or flexible? "skeletons in he closet"?

(Personal) Power: Emphasize What aspect of your life needs emphasis? What's neglected?

Faith/World View: Late Maturity/Death or **Reintegrative/Universalizing Faith**
Is it time to let go of concern for personal success, failure, contradiction, or injustice and simply concentrate on the greater good, or do you need be proactive in your own interests?

KIDNEY MERIDIAN FUNCTION	5-7 PM

Do you have vitality for growth and development, or are you operating on reserve energy/ just surviving? Drinking water, or purifying spiritually, emotionally, mentally, etc.?

PSOAS: What are you kicking? What paradox is in your life? What do you need to "sit up" and notice?

UPPER TRAPEZIUS: Is your head on straight? Do you have difficulty "seeing straight"?

ILIACUS: Is there something that needs to be kicked aside, or do you feel kicked aside?

 |

KIDNEY: 5-7 PM

Psoas: E, A, Water
Upper Trapezius: A, B, F, G, Calcium
Iliacus: Chlorophyll

162 C7

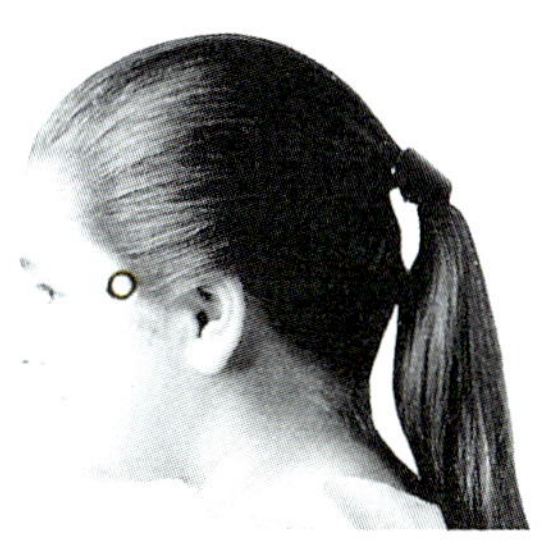

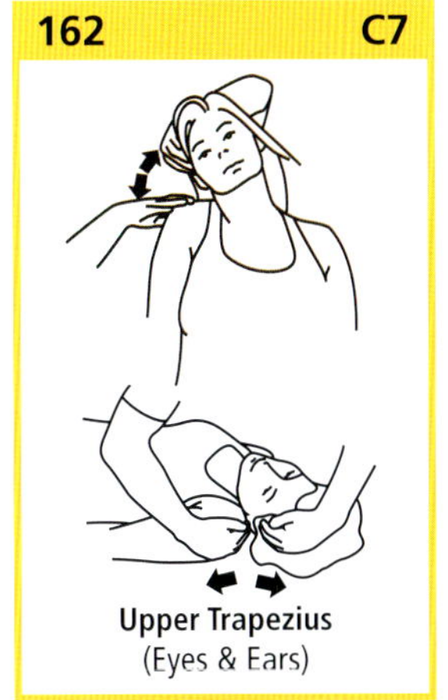

Upper Trapezius
(Eyes & Ears)

164 T11

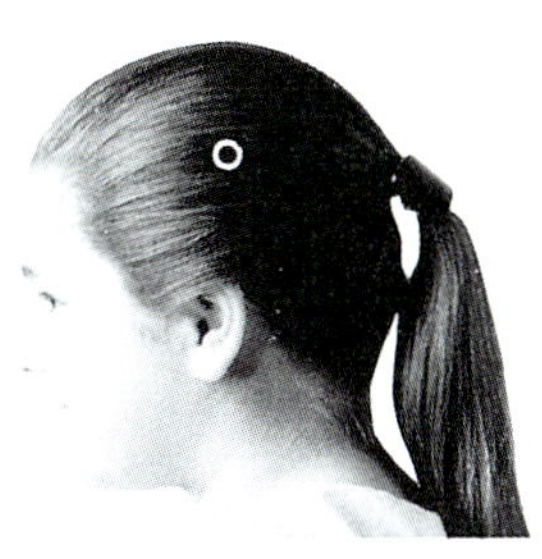

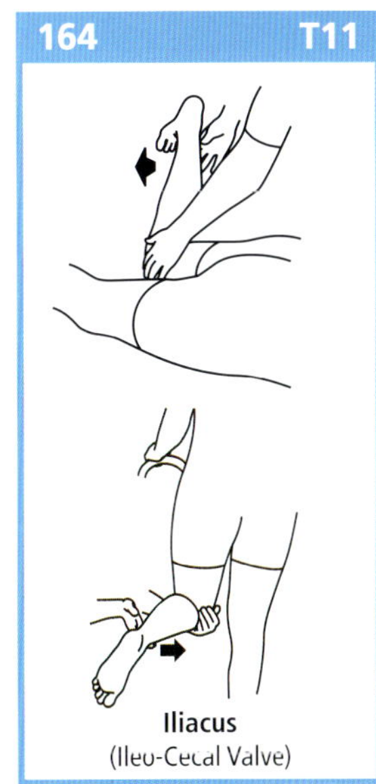

Iliacus
(Ileo-Cecal Valve)

Upper Trapezius
Psoas
Iliacus
T 12-L 1
A
A
Spinal Reflex Point
Alarm Point

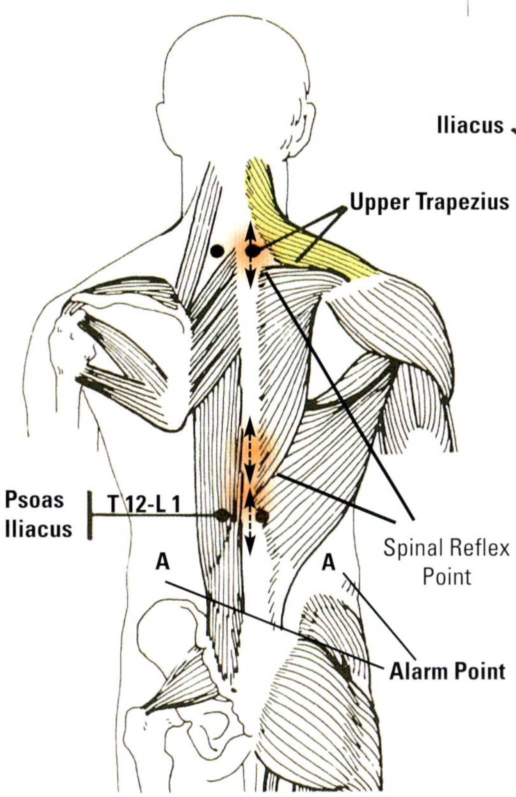

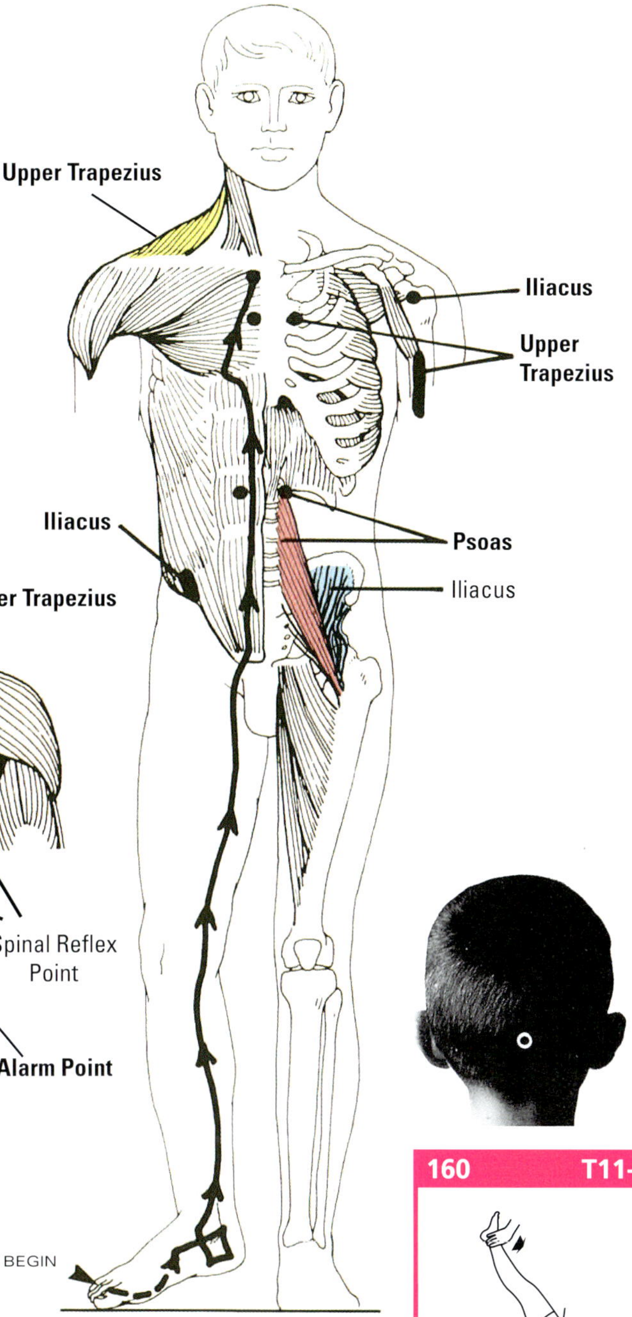

Upper Trapezius
Iliacus
Upper Trapezius
Iliacus
Psoas
Iliacus
BEGIN

160 T11-12

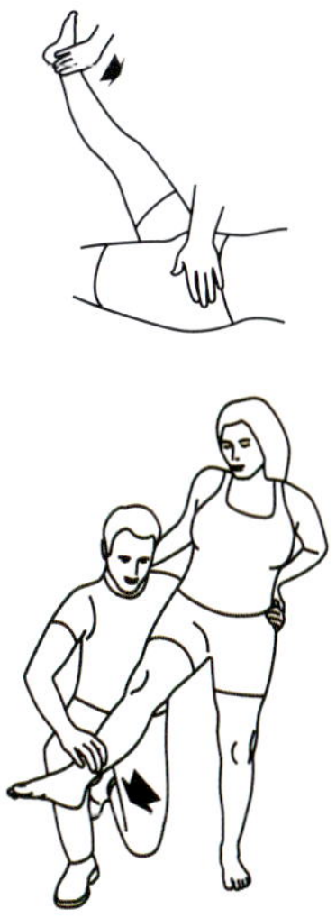

Psoas

ACUPRESSURE HOLDING POINTS

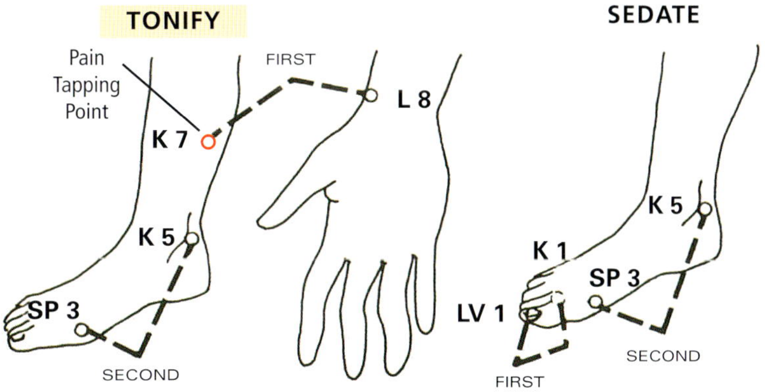

TONIFY
Pain Tapping Point
FIRST
L 8
K 7
K 5
SP 3
SECOND
SEDATE
K 5
K 1
SP 3
LV 1
SECOND
FIRST

THE FIRE ELEMENT

Heat, Burning, Energy, Passion, Action, Stimulation, Challenges, Danger

Do you have "fire in the belly", passion and energy for life? Are you too passionate, burning up your energy stores, burning those around you, or are you too cold, and unable to be passionate?

Color:Red Do you have enough Red in your life, or too much Red? Red alert?

Season: Summer Do you have "fun in the sun", or are you sensitive to light, sapped of energy?

Climate: Heat Can you take the Heat, or is the stress and pressure overwhelming? Are you too passionate, playing it too cool, or getting burned out? Do you run Hot or Cold? Need excitement?

Odor: Scorched Are you scorched by the elements, traumatic experiences, the passions, demands, or criticisms of others? Do you take risks, even at the cost of getting scorched? Smell danger?

Taste: Bitter What are your regrets or grudges? What's poisoning you? Too much stimulation, or not?

Emotion: Joy Do you need more Love and Joy in your life? Masking pain with a manic attitude/ drugs?

Sound: Laughing Do you enjoy mirth and Laughter. Avoid experiencing emotions by "laughing them off"? Have you laughed at the wrong moment? Been made fun of, laughed at, scorned or ridiculed?

Fortifies: Arteries Do you have a steady flow and distribution of the fuels and supplies to maintain your mental, emotional, spiritual and physical vitality? Does some part get poor circulation and go cold?

(Personal) Power: Mature Are you at ease with your limitations? Do you make full use of your capacities? Are you capricious? Do you experience childlike wonder and joy in life?

Faith/Worldview: Childhood/"School Years" or **Literal/Mythic Faith** Do you have a narrow, literal interpretation of rules, morals or beliefs? Are you conscious of conventions? Are you "re-inventing the wheel", "going it alone"? Do you expect precise reciprocity from others? Playing "tit for tat"?

CIRCULATION-SEX MERIDIAN FUNCTION	7-9 PM

How do you feel about reproduction and sex? Are you creating a legacy in your family, work, play, spiritual community? Do you have circulation of blood, warmth, nutrition or (sexual) energy? (also Pericardium) Do you support and protect your Heart?

GLUTEUS MEDIUS: What little things are you tripping over or bumping into? Are you "side-stepping"? Do you have any difficulty holding your legs open, literally or figuratively?

ADDUCTORS: Are you comfortable in the saddle, or saddle sore? Need to share or keep privacy?

PIRIFORMIS: Feeling knock-kneed, or clumsy? What small, subtle or deep issue is irritating you?

GLUTEUS MAXIMUS: Do you use your gross power to maintain overall stability or rely on strength when subtlety is needed? Are your sexual urges giving you a pain in the neck OR is your "head" (thinking) interfering with physical/survival/procreative needs?

 |

CIRCULATION-SEX: 7-9 PM | All Muscles: E

172 L1

Adductors

176 C2

Gluteus Maximus

To reach front Neuro Lymphatics move pectoralis up.

Alarm Point

BEGIN

A

Adductors

Pubic Bone

Gluteus Med.

Spinal Reflex Point

8-9

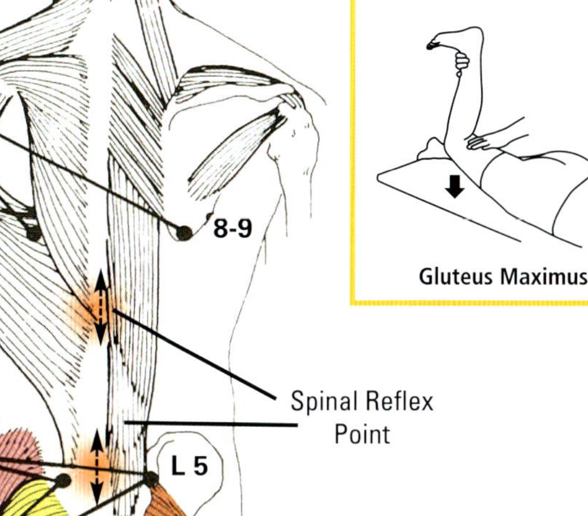

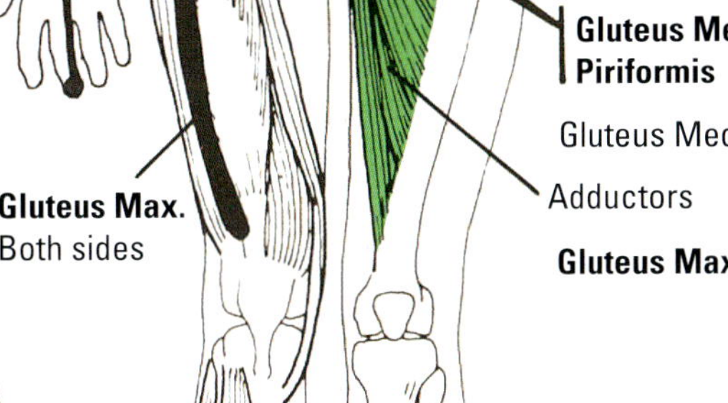

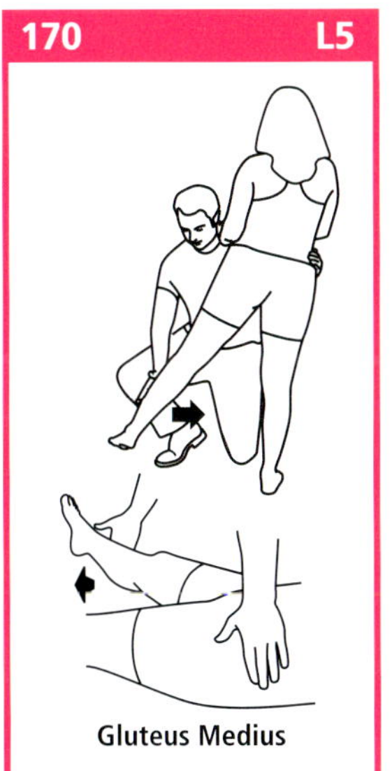

Gluteus Medius

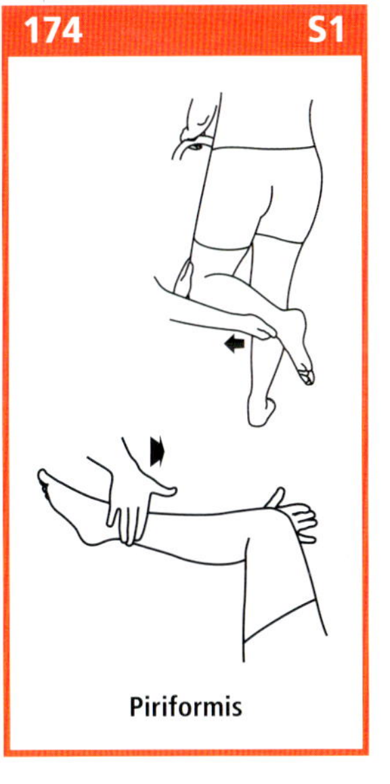

Piriformis

ACUPRESSURE HOLDING POINTS

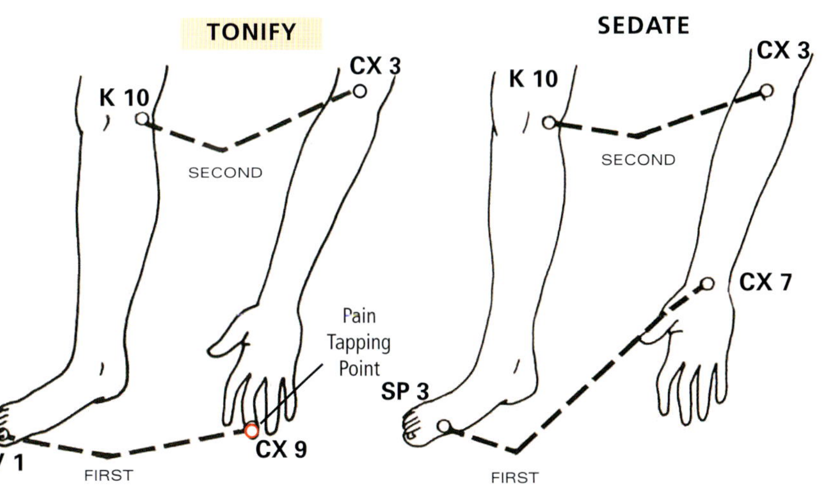

THE FIRE ELEMENT

Heat, Burning, Energy, Passion, Action, Stimulation, Challenges, Danger

Do you have "fire in the belly", passion and energy for life? Are you too passionate, burning up your energy stores, burning those around you, or are you too cold, and unable to be passionate?

Color:Red Do you have enough Red in your life, or too much Red? Red alert?

Season: Summer Do you have "fun in the sun", or are you sensitive to light, sapped of energy?

Climate: Heat Can you take the Heat, or is the stress and pressure overwhelming? Are you too passionate, playing it too cool, or getting burned out? Do you run Hot or Cold? Need excitement?

Odor: Scorched Are you scorched by the elements, traumatic experiences, the passions, demands, or criticisms of others? Do you take risks, even at the cost of getting scorched? Smell danger?

Taste: Bitter What are your regrets or grudges? What's poisoning you? Too much stimulation, or not?

Emotion: Joy Do you need more Love and Joy in your life? Masking pain with a manic attitude/ drugs?

Sound: Laughing Do you enjoy mirth and Laughter. Avoid experiencing emotions by "laughing them off"? Have you laughed at the wrong moment? Been made fun of, laughed at, scorned or ridiculed?

Fortifies: Arteries Do you have a steady flow and distribution of the fuels and supplies to maintain your mental, emotional, spiritual and physical vitality? Does some part get poor circulation and go cold?

(Personal) Power: Mature Are you at ease with your limitations? Do you make full use of your capacities? Are you capricious? Do you experience childlike wonder and joy in life?

Faith/Worldview: Childhood/"School Years" or **Literal/Mythic Faith** Do you have a narrow, literal interpretation of rules, morals or beliefs? Are you conscious of conventions? Are you "re-inventing the wheel", "going it alone"? Do you expect precise reciprocity from others? Playing "tit for tat"?

TRIPLE WARMER MERIDIAN FUNCTION | 9-11 PM

What gets you hot, physically, mentally, spiritually or emotionally? Are you constantly fighting or always on the run? What are you willing to suffer/die for?

TERES MINOR: Do you need to open your arms to receive or are you trying to take in too much?

SARTORIUS: Do you have the strength or passion to "go the distance", or to give your all?

GRACILIS: Do you feel clumsy or shy about passions? Do your passions get out of your control?

SOLEUS: Know when to stand and fight or retreat? Are you unnecessarily aggressive, or fearful?

GASTROCNEMIUS:What are you running to or from? Do you "rise to the occasion"? Is life a crisis, or an endless series of crises?

 |

TRIPLE WARMER: 9-11 PM

Teres Minor: Iodine
Sartorius, Gracilis, Gastrocnemius, Soleus: C

184 T11

Sartorius (Adrenal)

186 T12

Gracilis (Adrenal)

190 T11-12

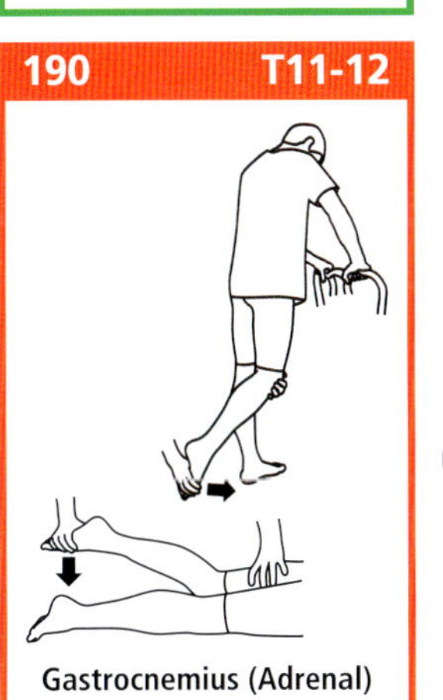

Gastrocnemius (Adrenal)

Spinal Reflex Point

2-3

Teres Minor

10-11

11-12

Sartorius
Gracilis
Gastroc.
Soleus

Both

2-3

A

Alarm Point

Sartorius

Gracilis

BEGIN

Gracilis

Gastrocnemius

Soleus

182 T2

Teres Minor (Thyroid)

188 T11-12

Soleus (Adrenal)

ACUPRESSURE HOLDING POINTS

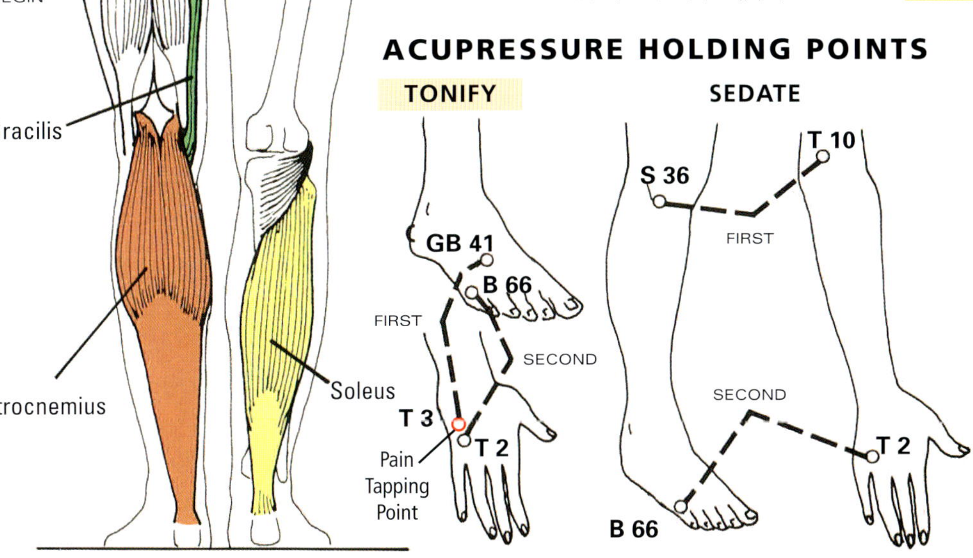

THE WOOD ELEMENT

New Beginnings, Vitality, Green Growth, Nature, Flexibility or Rigidity

Do you have enough roots, structure, and stability to sustain your growth? Do you need more freedom?

Color: Green Is there enough new growth? Are there more new ideas, projects than can be sustained?

Season: Spring What needs to be revived, renewed, or reborn? What seeds do you need to plant?

Climate: Wind Need "a breath of fresh air, a Spring Cleaning? Blown away by uncertainty and change?

Odor: Rancid Feeling stagnant physically, emotionally, mentally or spiritually? What's gone Rancid?

Taste: Sour Has something that was good gone bad? Do you need to make lemons into lemonade?

Emotion: Anger Directed appropriately (self, others, etc.)? *Can* you feel outrage, or passions in general?

Sound: Shouting Need to shout/voice your feelings and ideas? Are you "blowing hot air" ?

Fortifies: Ligaments Do you take precautions? "Push the envelope"? Run on reserves, overextend?

(Personal) PowerBirth: What do you need to give birth to? Need a fresh start? Starting too much?

Worldview/Faith: Infancy/Early Childhood or **Intuitive-Projective Faith** Is there only one correct viewpoint? Do you use personal intuition, and dream imagery to find meaning? Are you dwelling in your own dream-world, ignoring cause and effect, assuming what is right for you will be accepted by others?

GALL BLADDER MERIDIAN FUNCTION | 11 PM TO 1 AM

Can you digest the heavy parts of your life? Are you too concentrated, needing dilution? Do you feel "gall", indignation? Are you surprised by the "nerve" of others?

ANTERIOR DELTOID: Are you able to "take care" of your head, or do you do things that result in headache. Are the heavy aspects of your life overwhelming you? Can you raise your arm, volunteer? Follow "Marching Orders"?

POPLITEUS: What subtle thing is a "pain in neck", interfering with your movements, literally or figuratively? Can you change course, "turn on a dime?"

 |

GALL BLADDER: 11 PM - 1 AM | Vitamin A

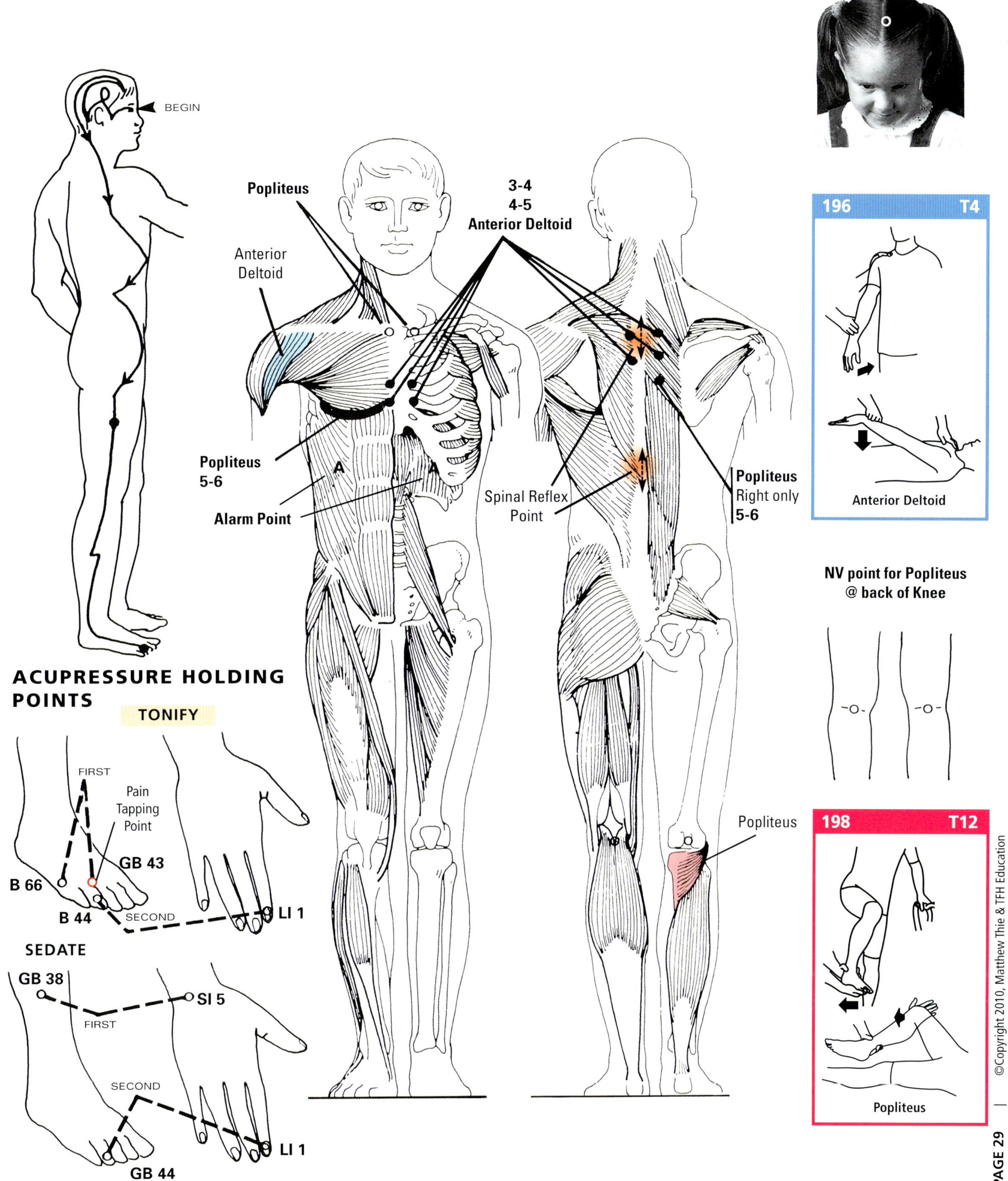

THE WOOD ELEMENT

New Beginnings, Vitality, Green Growth, Nature, Flexibility or Rigidity

Do you have enough roots, structure, and stability to sustain your growth? Do you need more freedom?

Color: Green Is there enough new growth? Are there more new ideas, projects than can be sustained?

Season: Spring What needs to be revived, renewed, or reborn? What seeds do you need to plant?

Climate: Wind Need "a breath of fresh air, a Spring Cleaning? Blown away by uncertainty and change?

Odor: Rancid Feeling stagnant physically, emotionally, mentally or spiritually? What's gone Rancid?

Taste: Sour Has something that was good gone bad? Do you need to make lemons into lemonade?

Emotion: Anger Directed appropriately (self, others, etc.)? *Can* you feel outrage, or passions in general?

Sound: Shouting Need to shout/voice your feelings and ideas? Are you "blowing hot air" ?

Fortifies: Ligaments Do you take precautions? "Push the envelope"? Run on reserves, overextend?

(Personal) PowerBirth: What do you need to give birth to? Need a fresh start? Starting too much?

Worldview/Faith: Infancy/Early Childhood or **Intuitive-Projective Faith** Is there only one correct viewpoint? Do you use personal intuition, and dream imagery to find meaning? Are you dwelling in your own dream-world, ignoring cause and effect, assuming what is right for you will be accepted by others?

LIVER MERIDIAN FUNCTION	1 TO 3 AM

How are you handling your multiple responsibilities? Are you overwhelmed/toxic, or do you need to absorb more? Are you missing resources or not processing well?

PECTORALIS MAJOR STERNAL: Are you too open? Need to harvest, collect or purify? Feel ALIVE and Vital?

RHOMBOIDS: Are you uptight/ posturally defensive? Holding on to toxins/ emotions? Need to open your chest?

 |

LIVER: 1-3 AM | A, F, Methionine

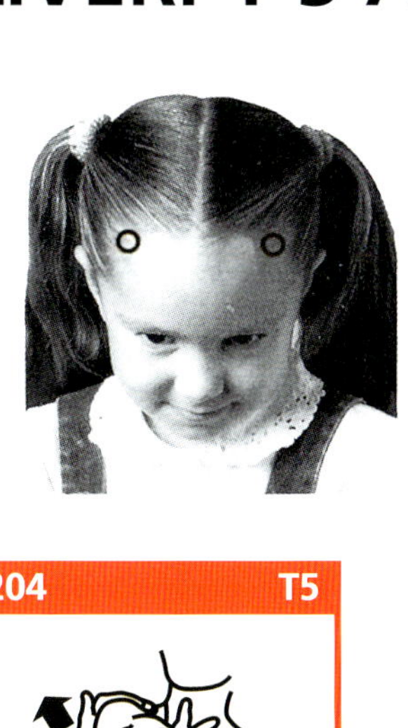

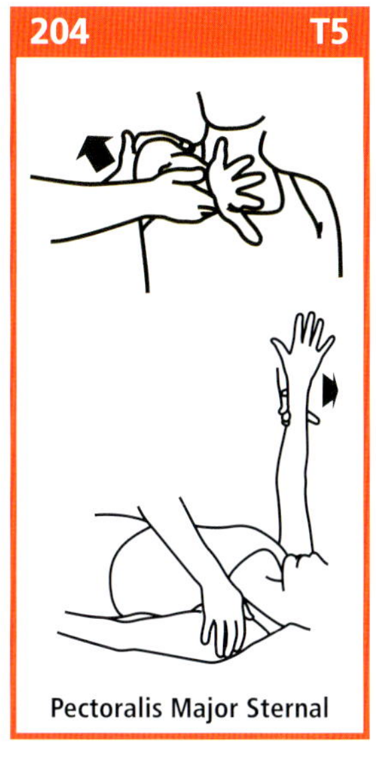

Pectoralis Major Sternal

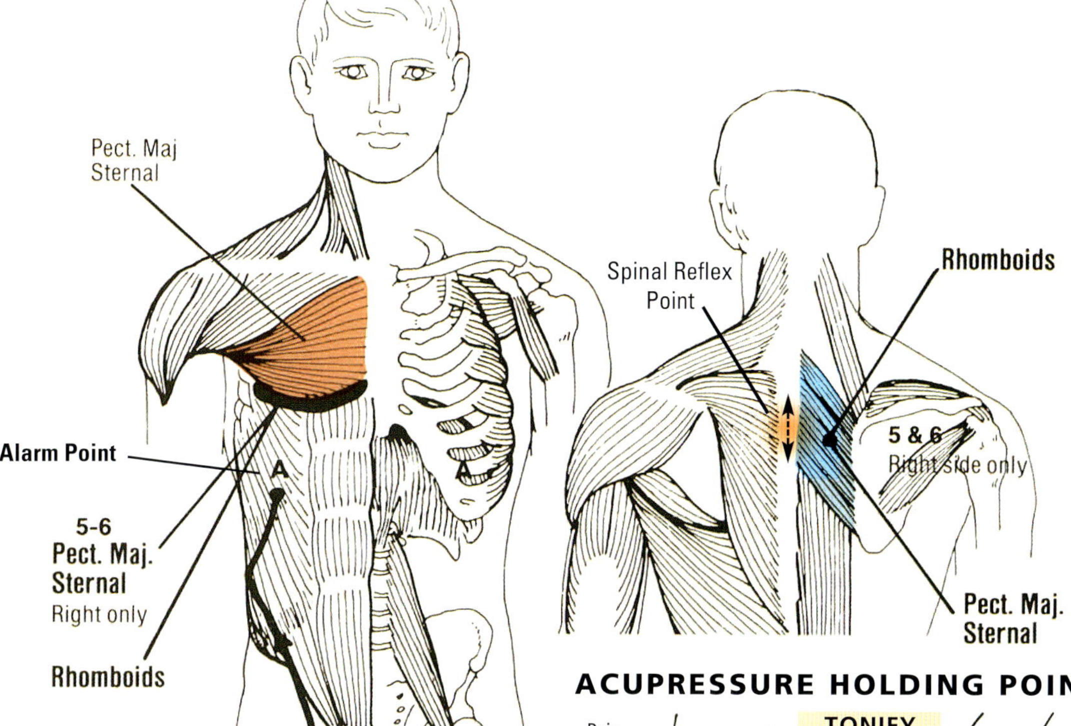

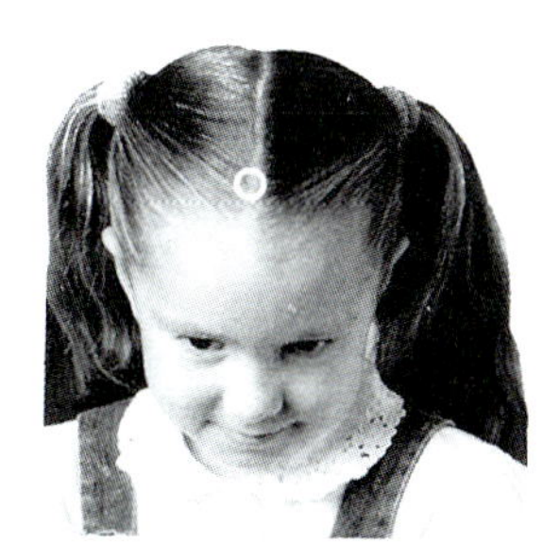

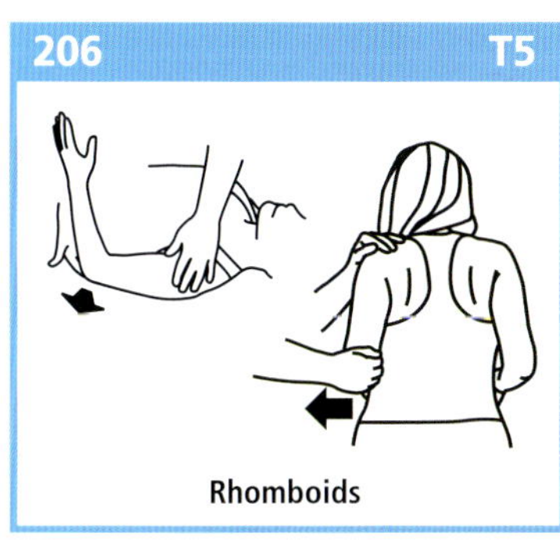

Rhomboids

ACUPRESSURE HOLDING POINTS

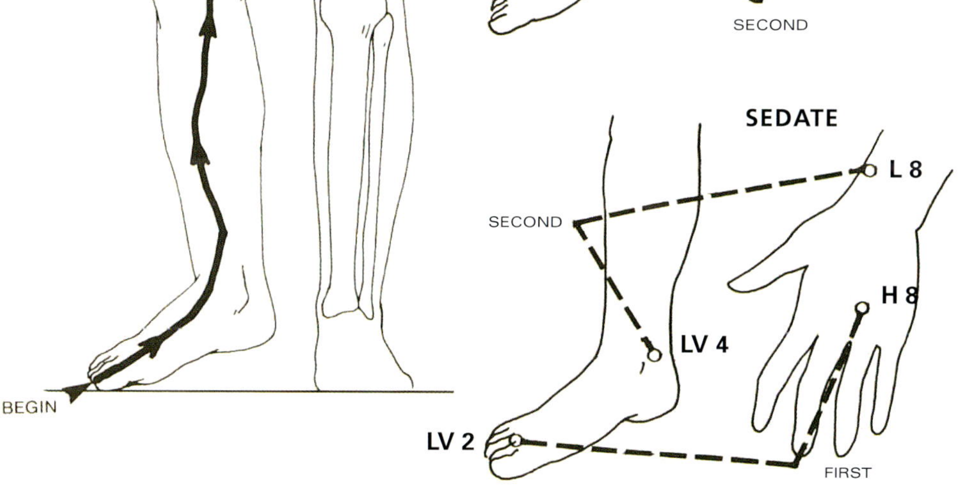

THE METAL ELEMENT

Armor/ Protection/ Weapons/ Tools
Adornment, Shiny Things, Money

Do you need a "hard shell", barriers or boundaries or do you need to open up more, let down your shield or mask?
Are you too hard or not hard enough on yourself or others?
Are you focused on adornment and appearances?
Need to pay some attention to how you present yourself?

Color: White Do you have pure light of truth or the mere appearance of truth: shiny things?

Season: Autumn Have you harvested the fruit of your labor, or has disaster/inattention spoiled it?

Climate: Dryness Do you need more moisture or a chance to "dry out"? Too dry, or too exciting?

Odor: Rotten What is rotten in your life? Have good things become corrupt, rotten, and wasted?

Taste: Pungent Is there enough spice in your life or is it too hot, painful or dangerous?

Emotion: Grief What have you lost or sacrificed /will lose (so that you can reach your goals)?

Sound: Weeping Do you hold it all in or do you cry when it's not appropriate?

Fortifies: Skin and Hair Are you "thin skinned" or "thick skinned"? Well groomed or not?

Personal Power: Balance What aspects of your life are out of balance? Is life static or stagnant?

Faith/Worldview: Young Adulthood or **Responsible Faith** Do you take personal responsibility for your beliefs and actions, or is life shaped by the roles you play and the meaning you have for others?

LUNG MERIDIAN FUNCTION	3 TO 5 AM

Can you breath/speak easily? Do you have a free flow of fresh air and inspiration or are you constricted, inhibited, literally/figuratively? Need to shout, cheer, or cough it up?

ANTERIOR SERRATUS: Lost your voice? Need to exert power, push, punch, or pushing too hard?

CORACOBRACHIALIS: Is it easy or painful to "take care of yourself"? Can you salute authority?

DELTOIDS: What needs uplifting? Do you give praise and receive inspiration, or do you feel stale?

DIAPHRAGM: Do you have fresh air? Can you breath, speak, or sing easily? Is your chest tight?

 |

LUNG: 3-5 AM | C, Water

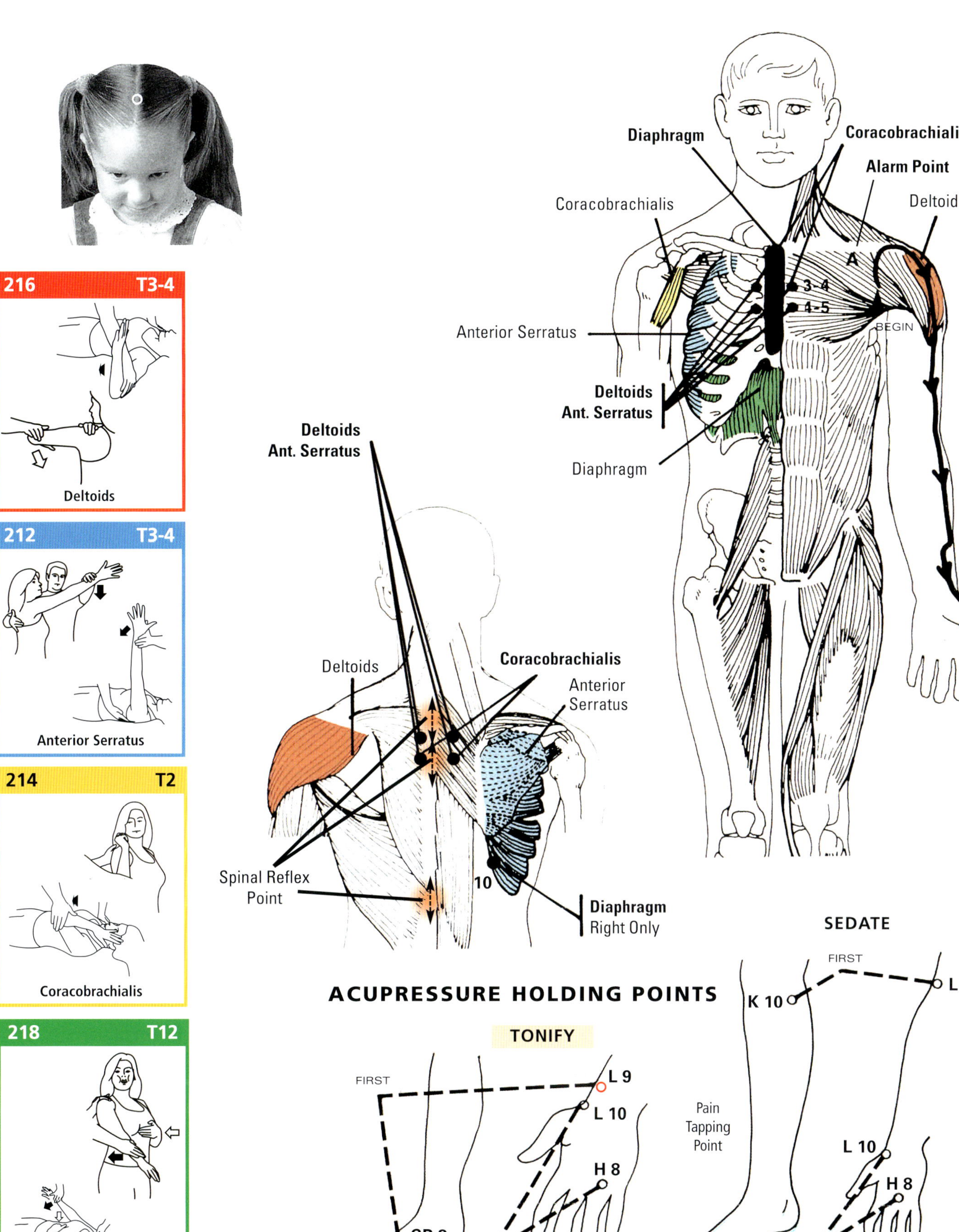

ACUPRESSURE HOLDING POINTS

THE METAL ELEMENT

Armor/ Protection/ Weapons/ Tools
Adornment, Shiny Things, Money

Do you need a "hard shell", barriers or boundaries or do you need to open up more, let down your shield or mask?
Are you too hard or not hard enough on yourself or others?
Are you focused on adornment and appearances?
Need to pay some attention to how you present yourself?

Color: White Do you have pure light of truth or the mere appearance of truth: shiny things?

Season: Autumn Have you harvested the fruit of your labor, or has disaster/inattention spoiled it?

Climate: Dryness Do you need more moisture or a chance to "dry out"? Too dry, or too exciting?

Odor: Rotten What is rotten in your life? Have good things become corrupt, rotten, and wasted?

Taste: Pungent Is there enough spice in your life or is it too hot, painful or dangerous?

Emotion: Grief What have you lost or sacrificed /will lose (so that you can reach your goals)?

Sound: Weeping Do you hold it all in or do you cry when it's not appropriate?

Fortifies: Skin and Hair Are you "thin skinned" or "thick skinned"? Well groomed or not?

Personal Power: Balance What aspects of your life are out of balance? Is life static or stagnant?

Faith/Worldview: Young Adulthood or **Responsible Faith** Do you take personal responsibility for your beliefs and actions, or is life shaped by the roles you play and the meaning you have for others?

LARGE INTESTINE MERIDIAN FUNCTION	5 TO 7 AM

Do you retain things you can no longer use (until they become toxic) or are you letting too much go? Can you identify what is valuable to keep and (re)integrate and what is trash or is not serving you?

FASCIA LATA: Do you feel that you have power and thrust in your walk (or race) of life?

HAMSTRINGS: Can you make changes while in full stride? Has a change caused strain or injury?

QUADRATUS LUMBORUM: Can you be upright? Are you flexible, physically, in work/life/goals?

 |

LARGE INTESTINE: 5-7 AM

Fascia Lata: Iron, B, Lactobacillus
Hamstrings: E
Quadratus Lumborum: E, A, C

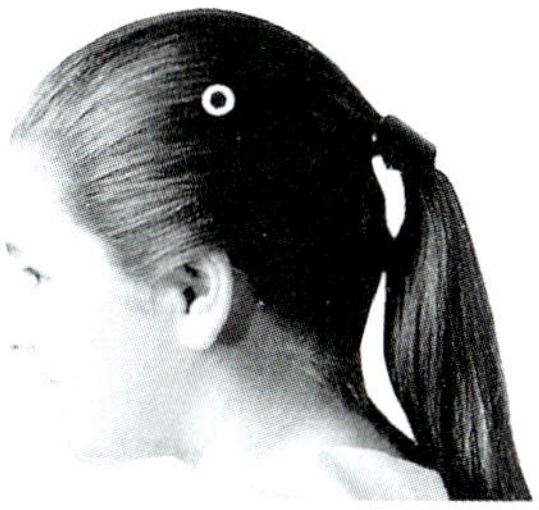

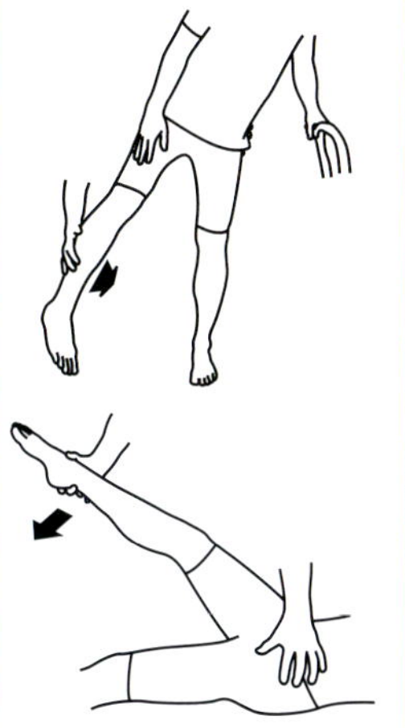

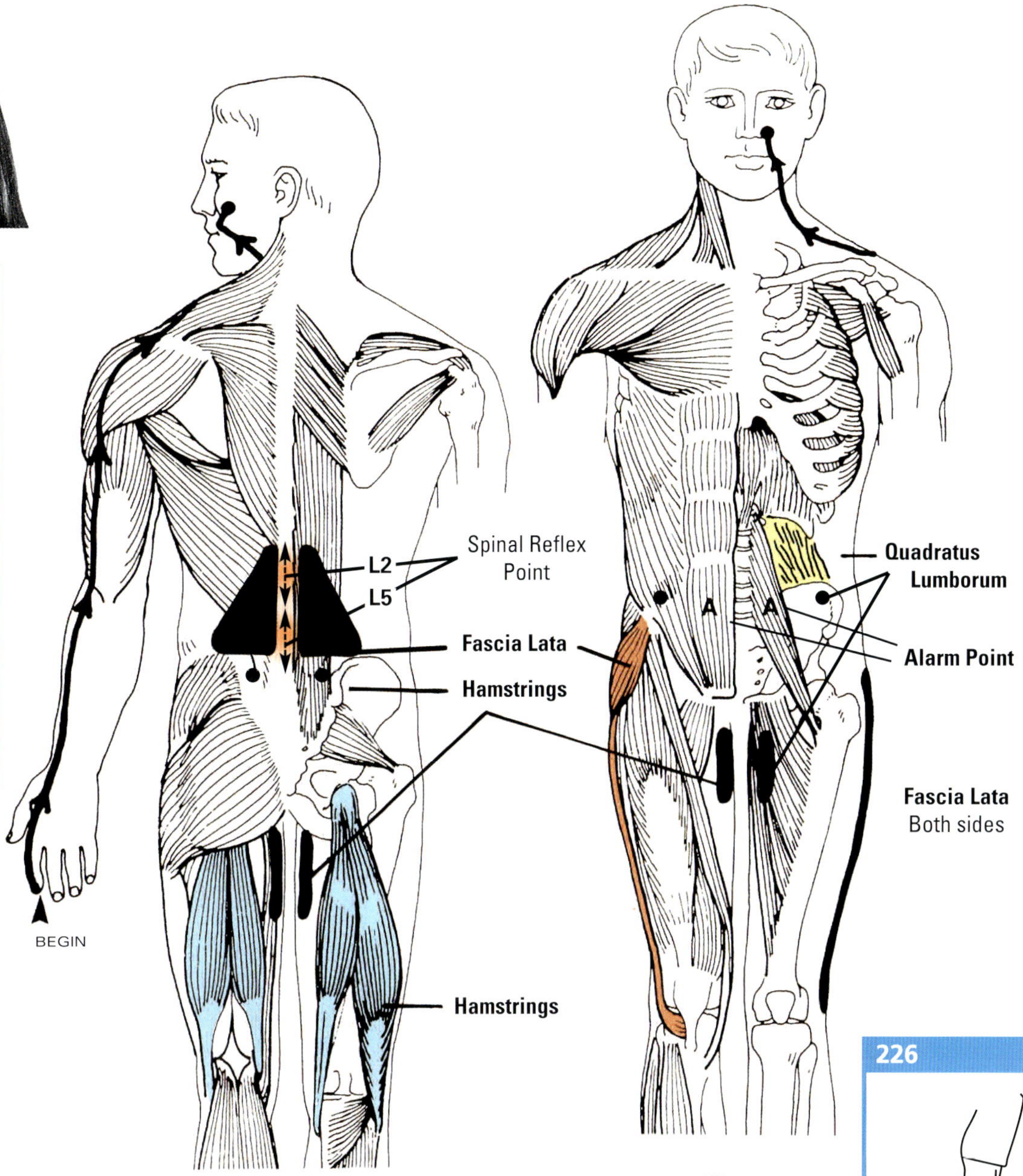

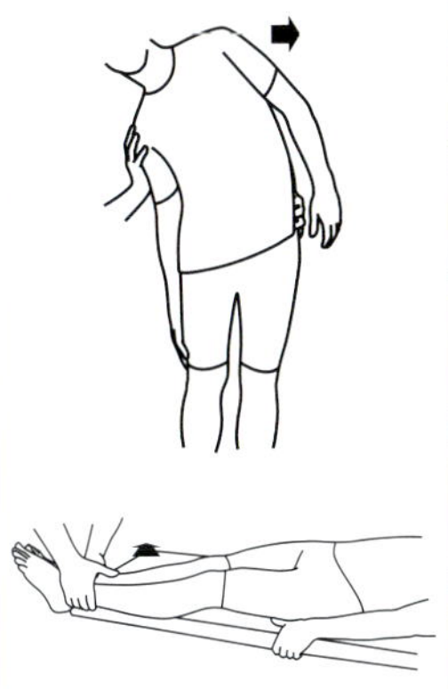

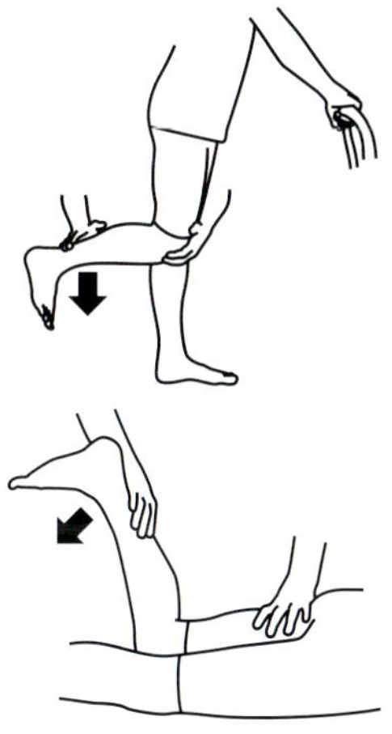

ACUPRESSURE HOLDING POINTS

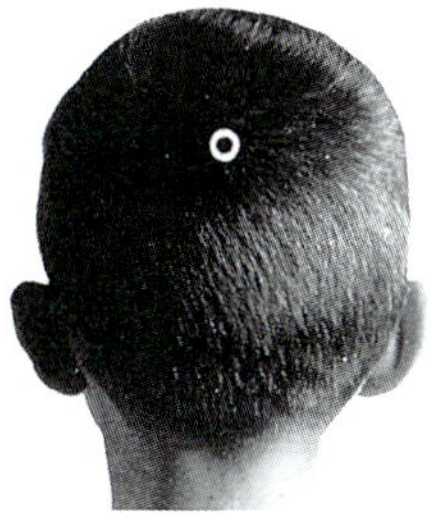

TONIFY

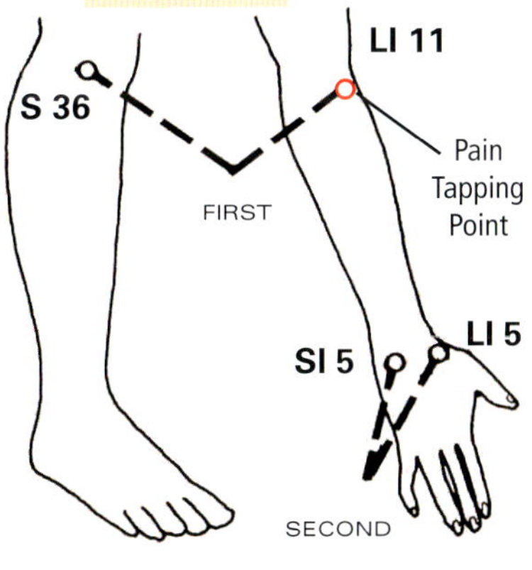

SEDATE

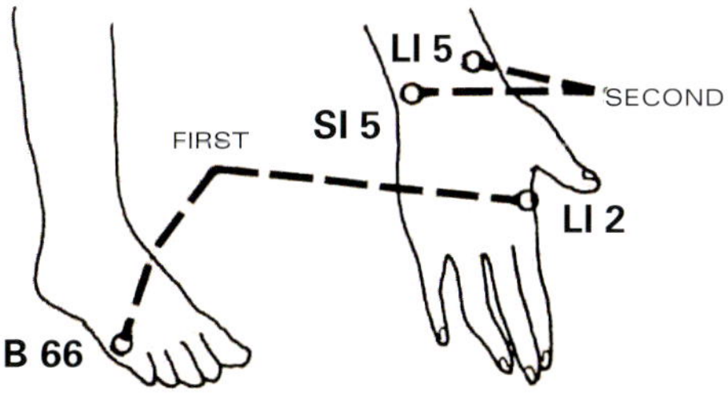

ELECTRICAL / ENERGETIC

MENTAL / EMOTIONAL

STRUCTURAL

REACTIVITY

 |

BIOCHEMICAL

PAIN CONTROL

* Please note that the 14-Meridian TFH balance has been found to be very effective for alleviating pain and other symptoms. Any balancing technique may also be employed for relief of pain. Circuit-Locate the entire database for other possibilities to try.

Use common sense & seek appropriate professional care for injuries, serious symptoms, or if symptoms continue or worsen after balancing. Pain relief does not necessarily mean resolution of a condition, so check with your doctor!

SUPPORT TECHNIQUES

ENERGY BALANCING TOUCH REFLEXES

 |

42 - MUSCLES HEAD TO TOE

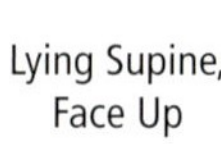

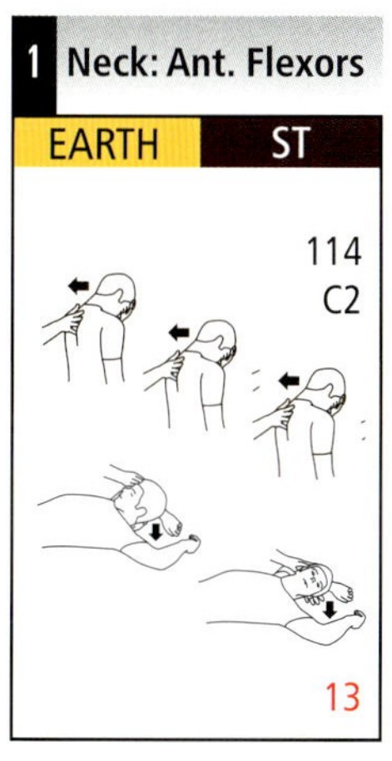

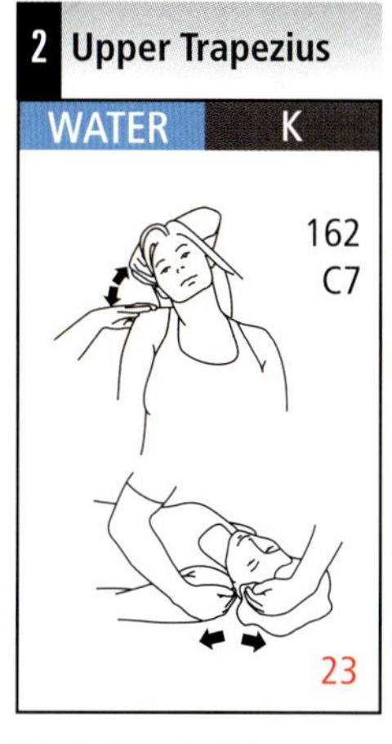

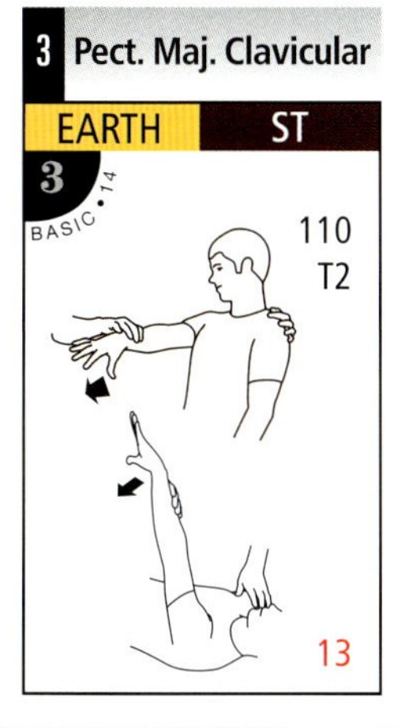

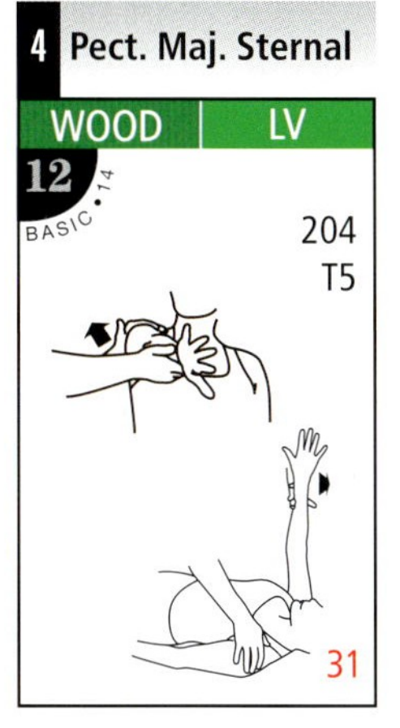

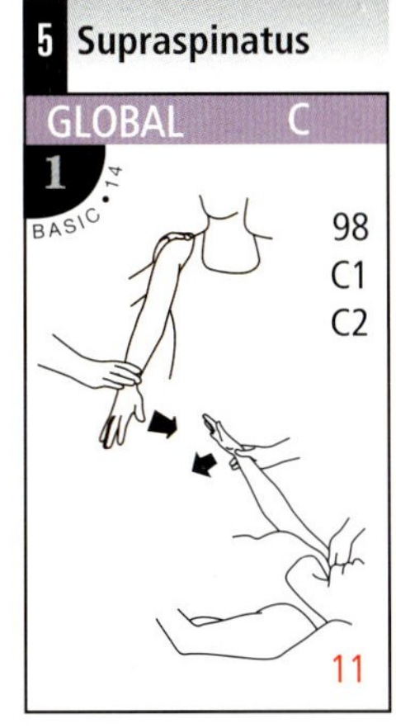

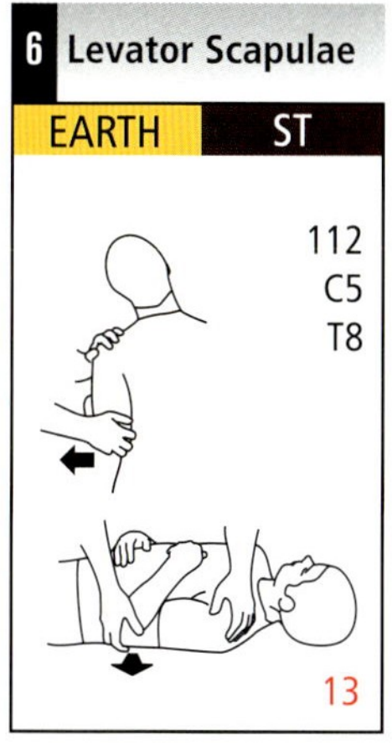

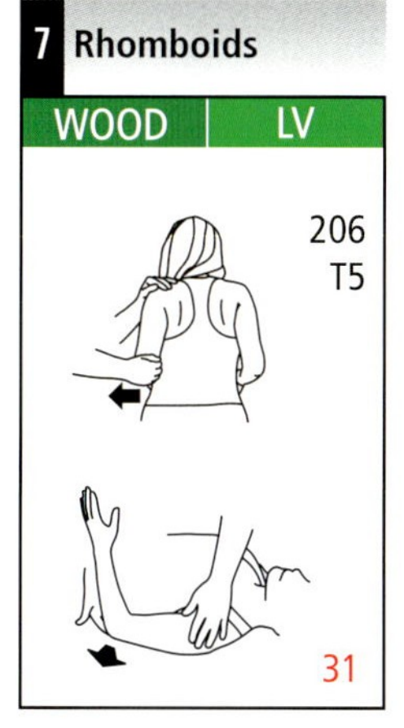

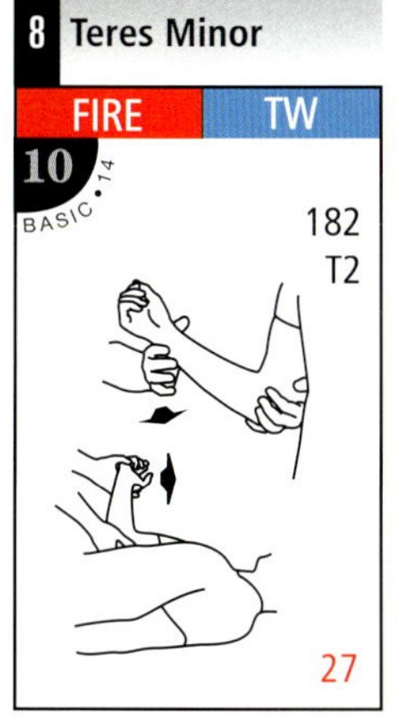

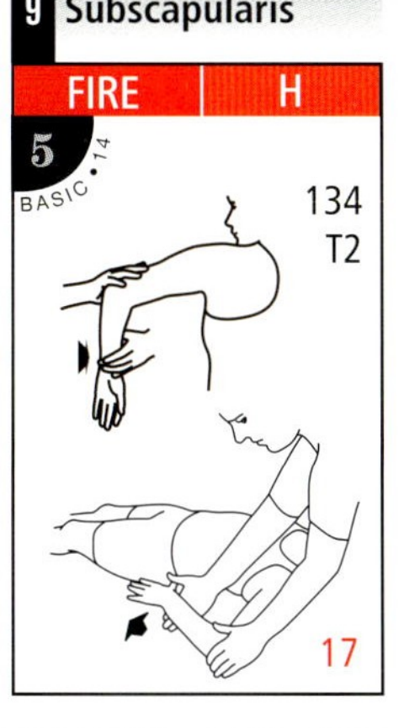

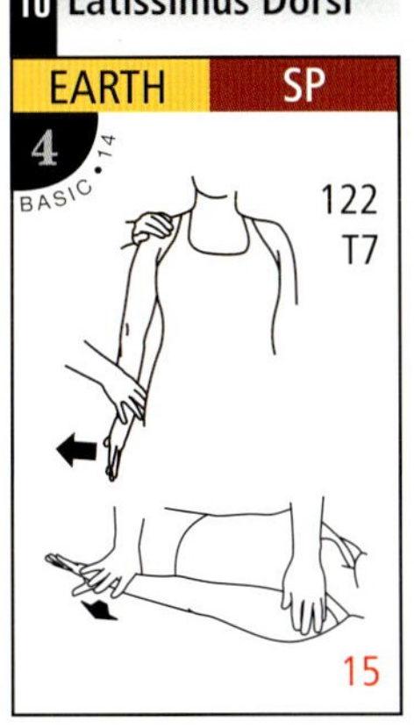

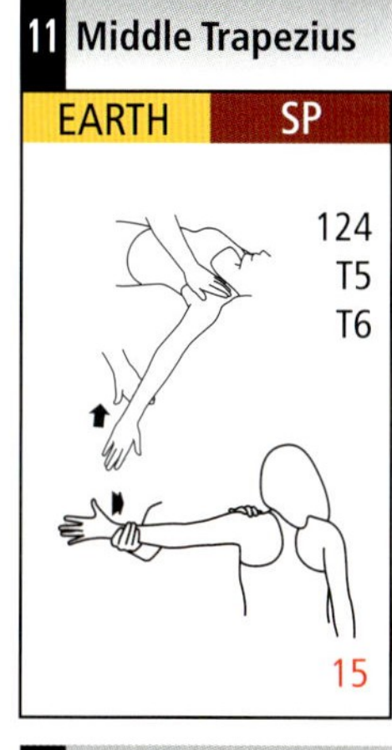

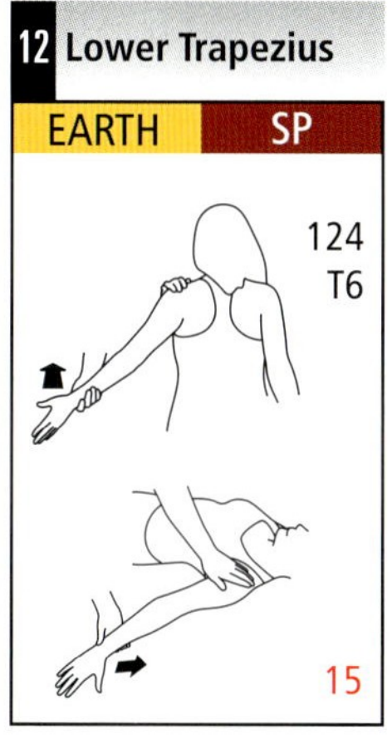

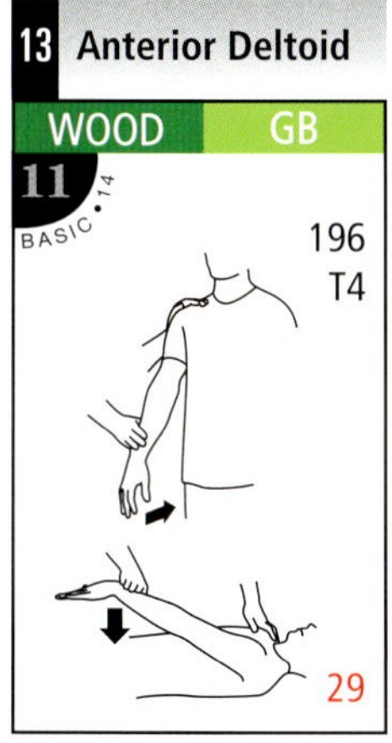

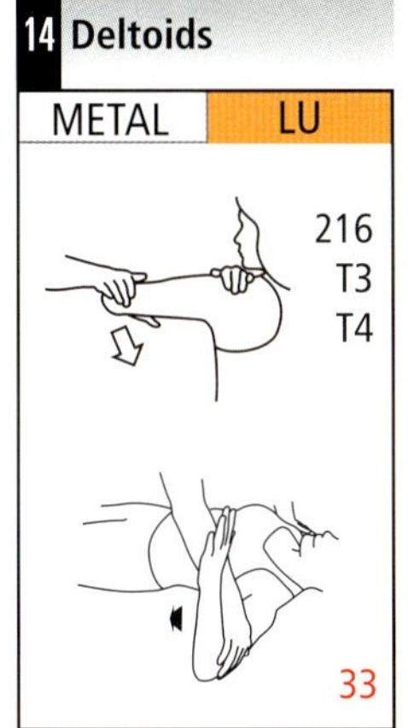

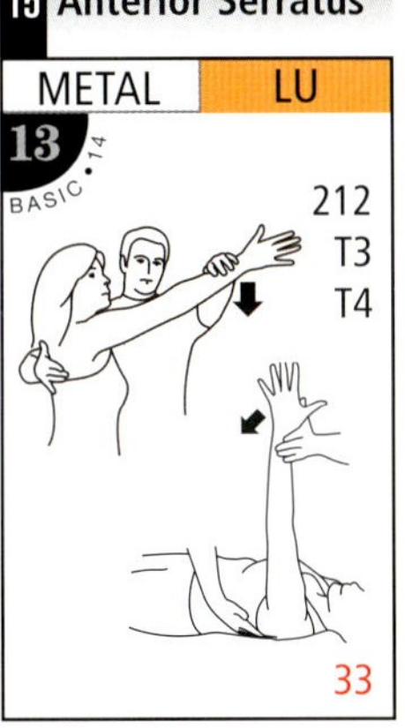

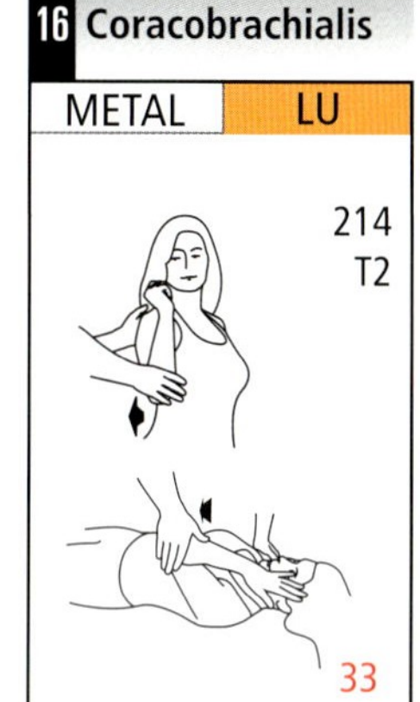

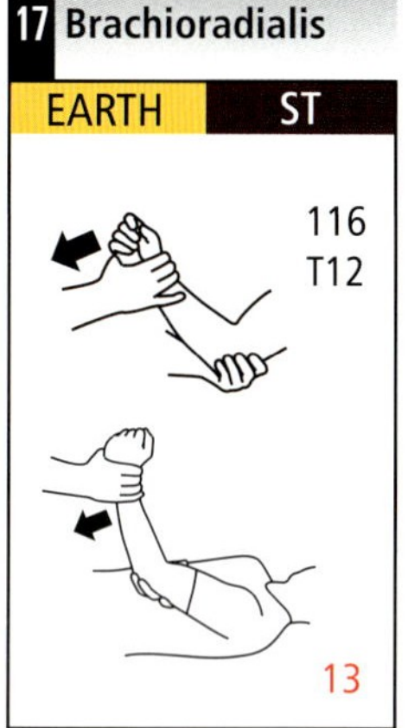

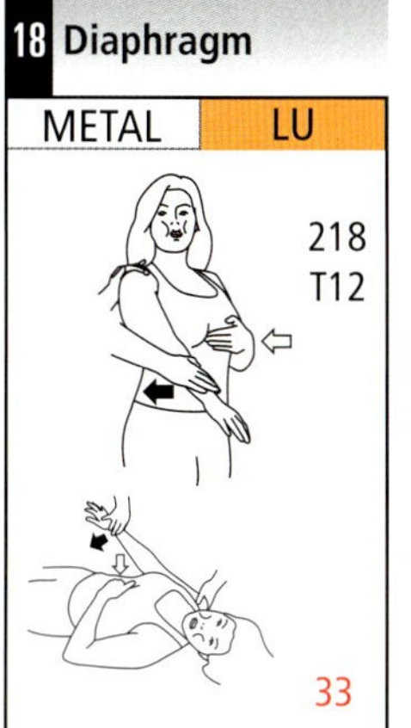

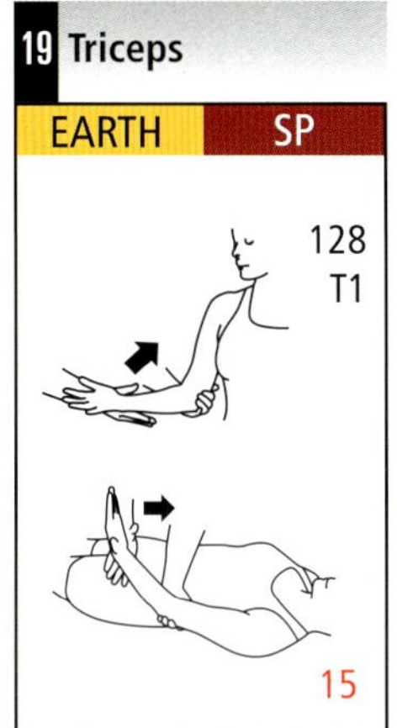

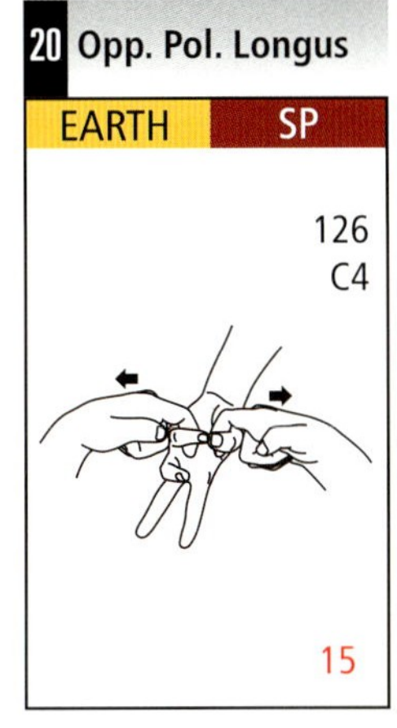

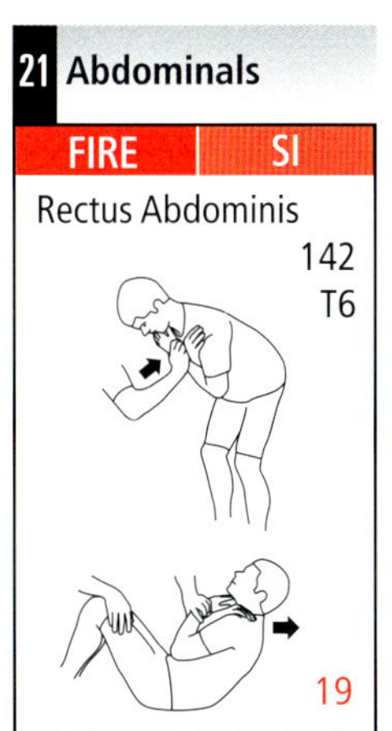

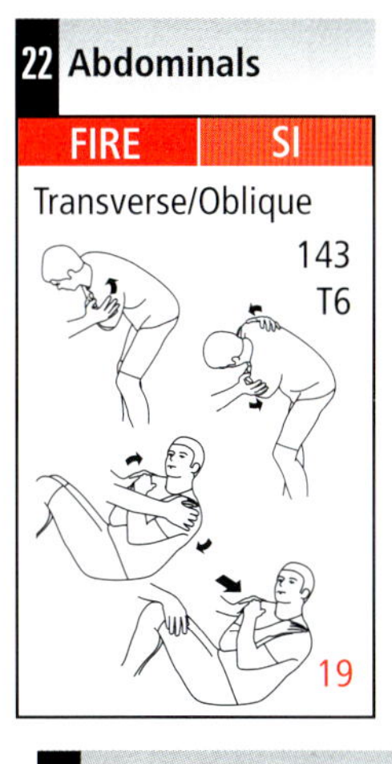

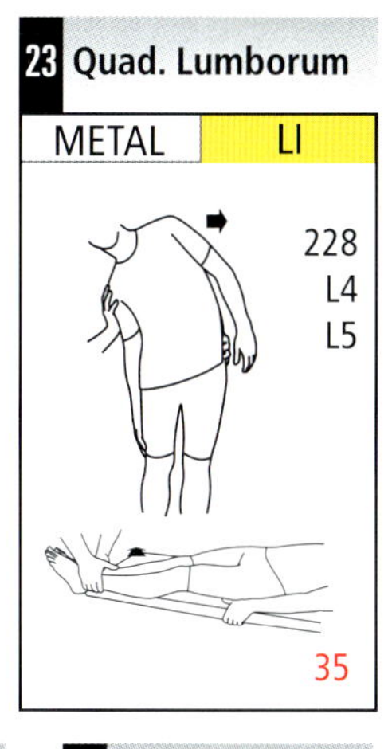

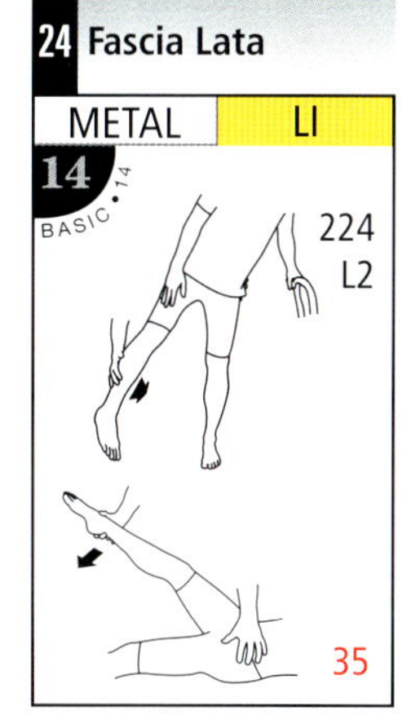

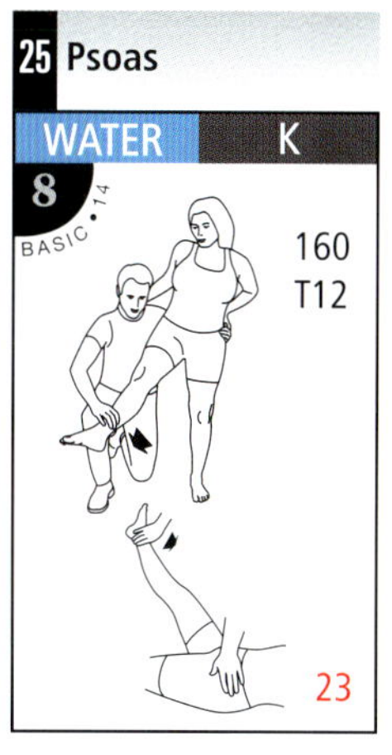

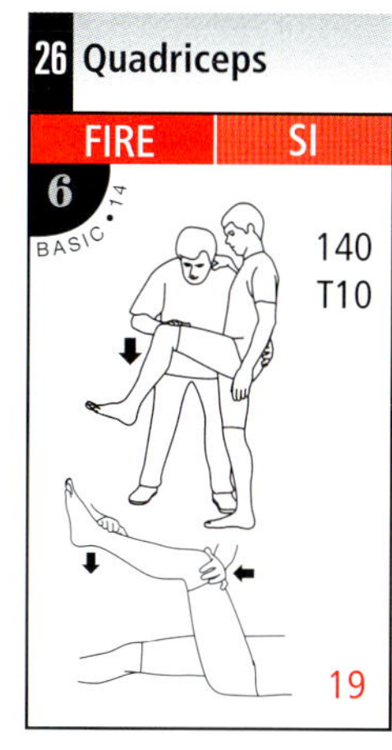

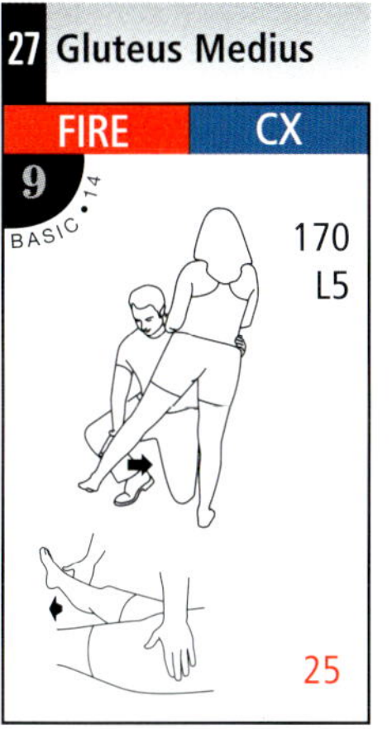

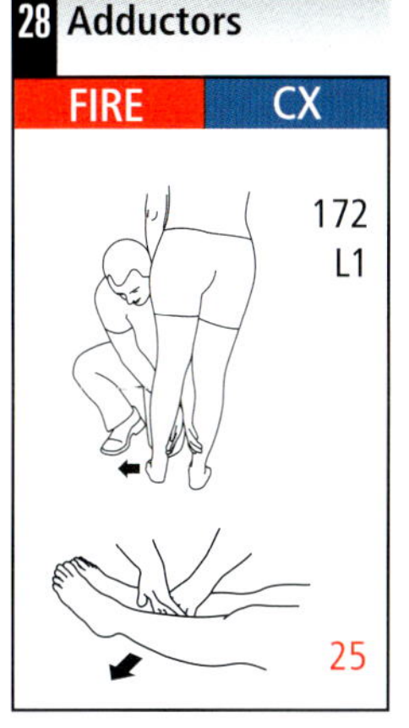

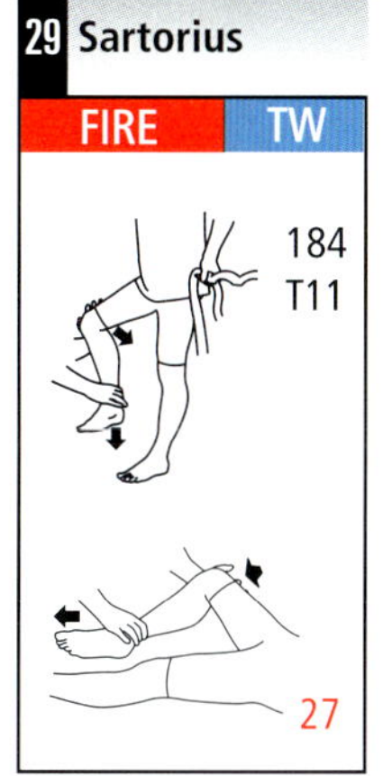

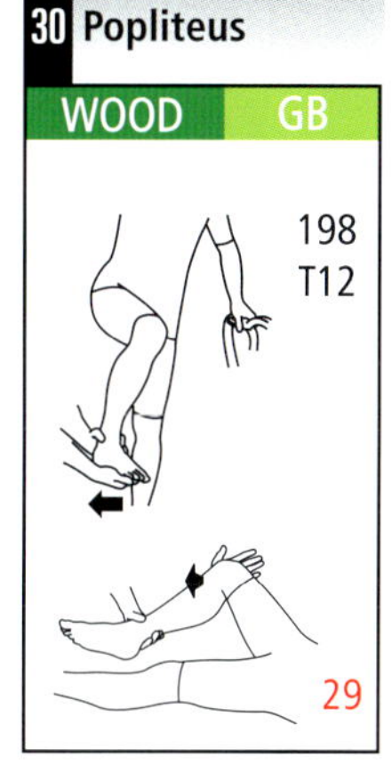

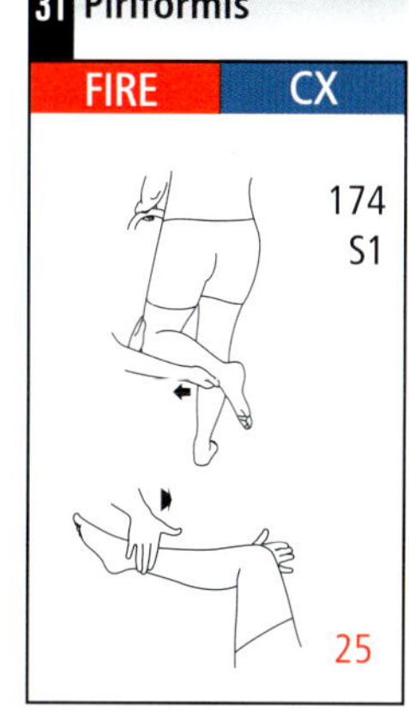

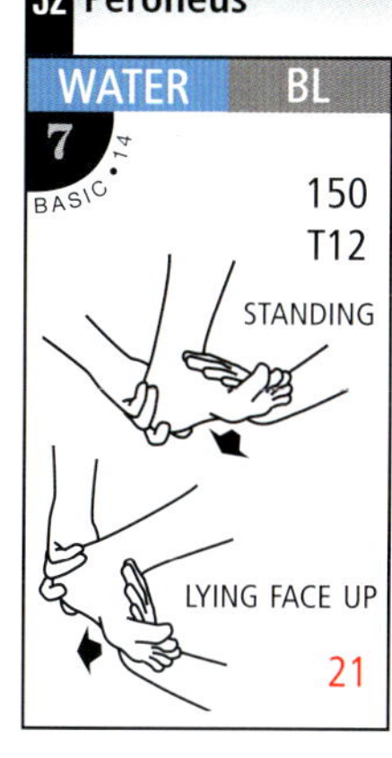

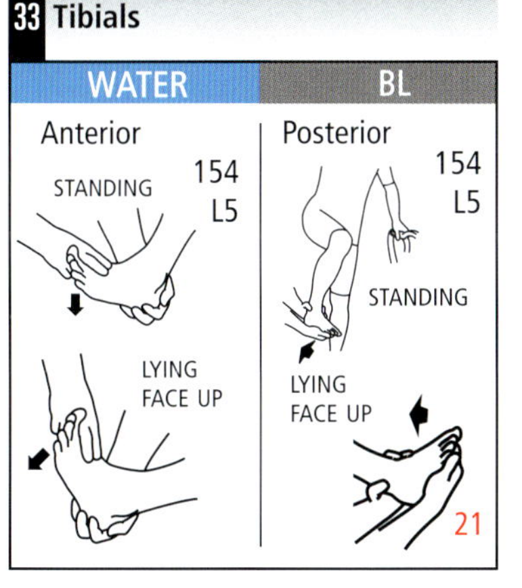

Turn Prone,
Face Down

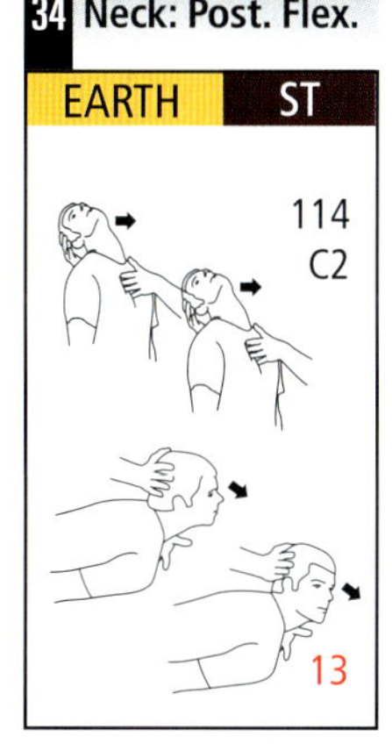

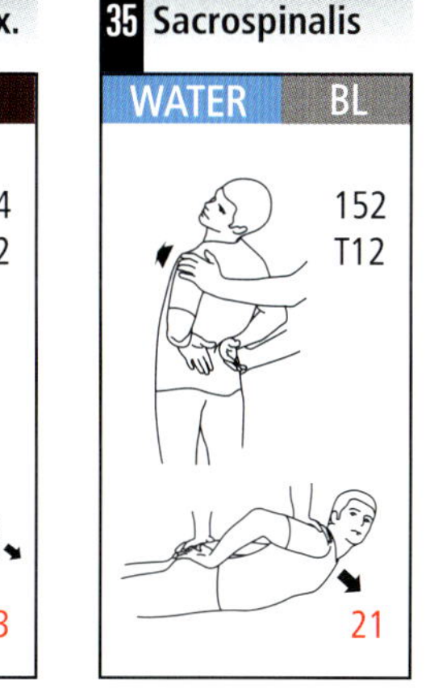

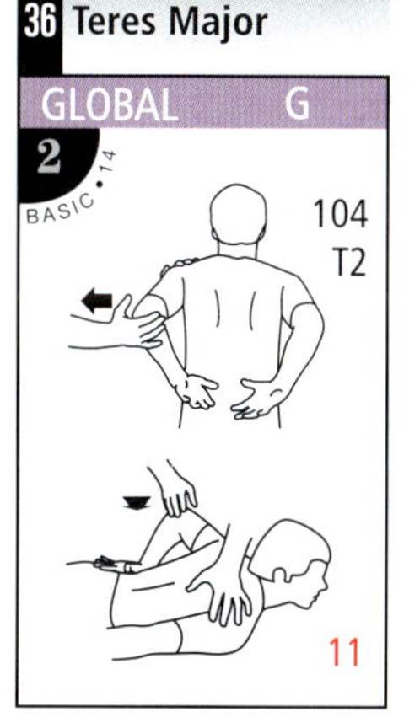

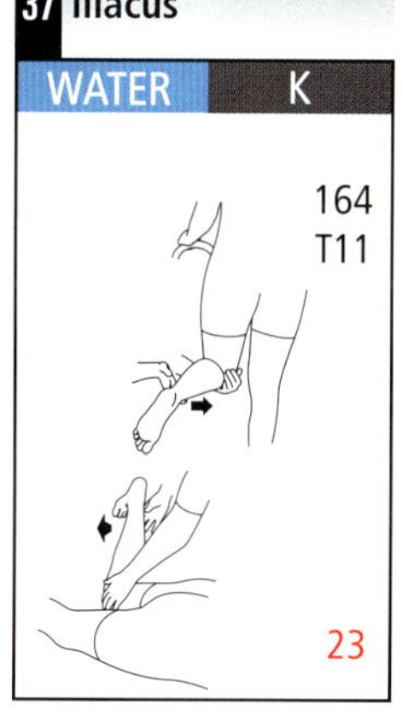

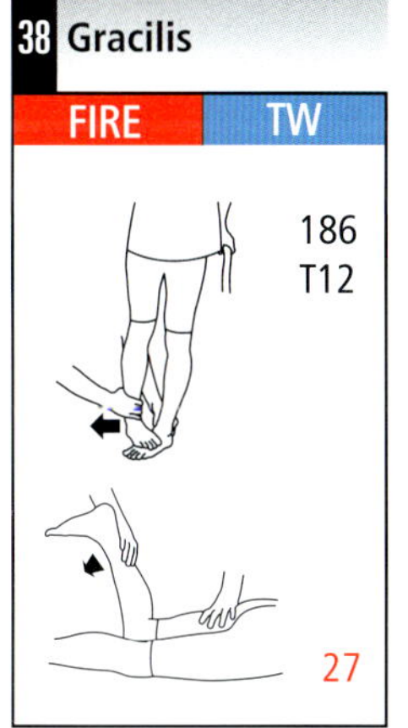

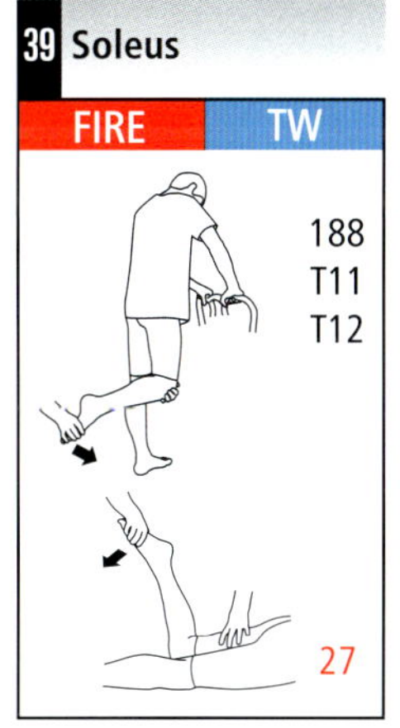

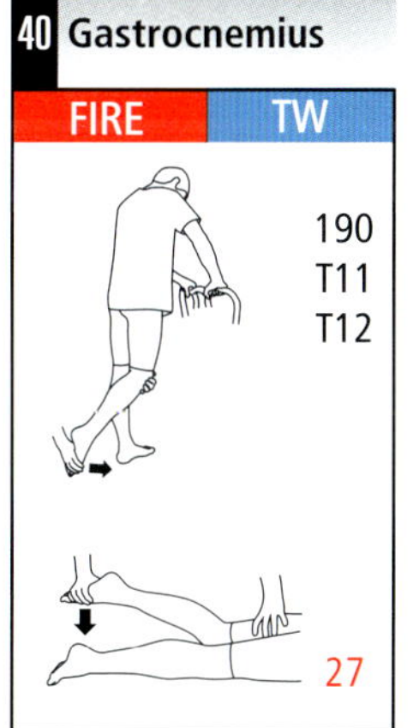

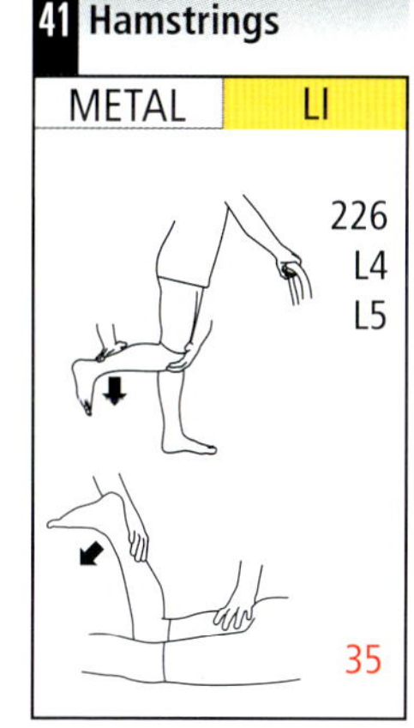

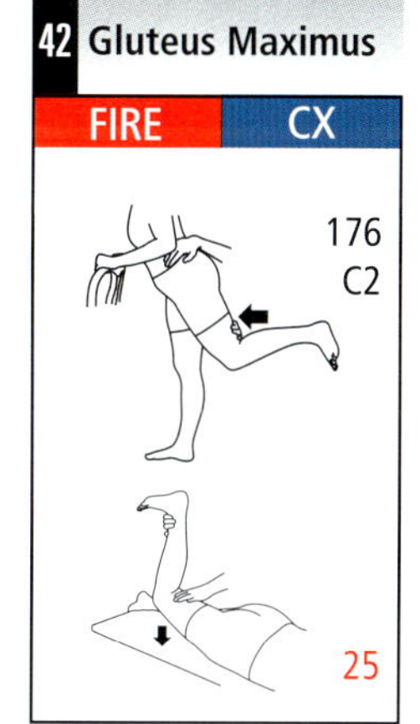

LUO POINTS

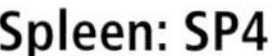

Spleen: SP4
On the Spleen Meridian, 4 body" from the nail root of the big toe and toward the ankle.

Stomach: ST40
On the Stomach Meridian, on the outside of the leg, midway between the anklebone and the kneecap.

Lung: LU7
On the Lung Meridian, 2 body" above the first crease on the wrist at the base of the hand.

Large Intestine: LI6
On the Large Intestine Meridian, 3 body"above the wrist crease at the base of the hand.

Kidney: K4
On the Kidney Meridian, on the inside of the leg level with the middle of the anklebone.

Bladder: BL58
On the Bladder Meridian, on the outside of the leg, near the bottom of Gastrocnemius (calf) muscle.

Liver: LV5
On the Liver Meridian, 5 body" above the inside anklebone.

Gallbladder: GB37
On the Gallbladder Meridian, 5 body" above the outside anklebone.

Heart: H5
On the Heart Meridian, 1 body" above the wrist crease at the base of the hand.

Small Intestine: SI7
On the Small Intestine Meridian, 5 body" above the wrist flexure, outside aspect of the arm.

Circulation-Sex: CX6
On the Circulation-Sex Meridian, 2 body" above the wrist crease at the base of the hand.

Triple Warmer: TW5
On the Triple Warmer Meridian, 2 body" above the crease on the backside of the wrist

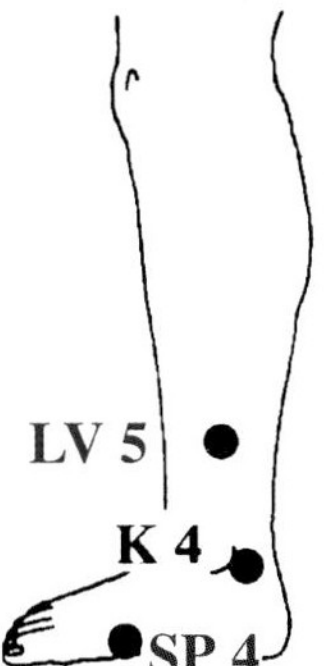

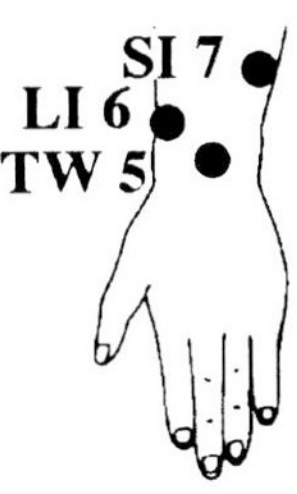

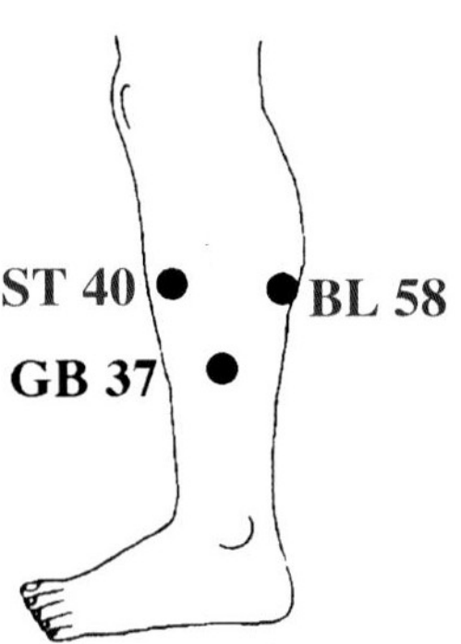

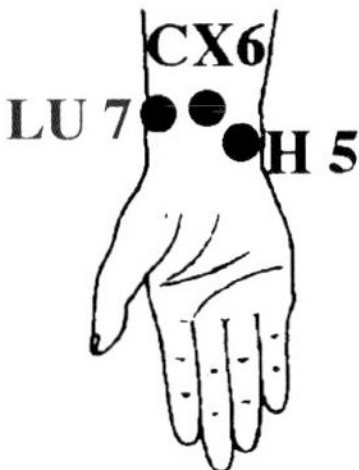

The Luo Points can all be found bilaterally.

Used with Permission, IKC Coursebook II, pg. 15.

